STRESS MANAGEMENT

Strategies and Techniques for Living a Healthy Life

(How to Stop Overthinking and How to Start Thinking Positively)

Meghan Smith

Published By Bengion Cosalas

Meghan Smith

All Rights Reserved

Stress Management: Strategies and Techniques for Living a Healthy Life (How to Stop Overthinking and How to Start Thinking Positively)

ISBN 978-1-77485-370-2

All rights reserved. No part of this guide may be reproduced in any form without permission in writing from the publisher except in the case of brief quotations embodied in critical articles or reviews.

Legal & Disclaimer

The information contained in this book is not designed to replace or take the place of any form of medicine or professional medical advice. The information in this book has been provided for educational and entertainment purposes only.

The information contained in this book has been compiled from sources deemed reliable, and it is accurate to the best of the Author's knowledge; however, the Author cannot guarantee its accuracy and validity and cannot be held liable for any errors or omissions. Changes are periodically made to this book. You must consult your doctor or get professional medical advice before using any of the suggested remedies, techniques, or information in this book.

Upon using the information contained in this book, you agree to hold harmless the Author from and against any damages, costs, and expenses, including any legal fees potentially resulting from the application of any of the information provided by this guide. This disclaimer applies to any damages or injury caused by the use and application, whether directly or indirectly, of any advice or information presented, whether for breach of contract, tort, negligence, personal injury, criminal intent, or under any other cause of action.

You agree to accept all risks of using the information presented inside this book. You need to consult a professional medical practitioner in order to ensure you are both able and healthy enough to participate in this program.

TABLE OF CONTENTS

INTRODUCTION 1

CHAPTER 1: WHAT IS STRESS MANAGEMENT? 4

CHAPTER 2: DEFINE SUCCESS 12

CHAPTER 3: THE TWO EXTREMES OF STRESS 23

CHAPTER 4: SYMPTOMS OF STRESS 43

CHAPTER 5: DEVELOP LONG-TERM RESILIENCE HABITS ... 47

CHAPTER 6: HABITS OF LIFE THAT EASE STRESS 67

CHAPTER 7: CONSIDERING THE LIFE CYCLE 72

CHAPTER 8: QUICK TIPS TO MANAGE STRESS 83

CHAPTER 9: RELAXATION TECHNIQUES 92

CHAPTER 10: SOCIAL STRESS 95

CHAPTER 11: THE WAY TO STOP SLEEPING WHILE THINKING 120

CHAPTER 12: MINDFULNESS MEDITATION 140

CHAPTER 13: STRESS MANAGEMENT FOR PARENTS 157

CHAPTER 14: THE DAILY AFFIRMATIONS 175

CONCLUSION 182

Introduction

The book is packed with practical steps and strategies to help you manage stress in the hope of improving your overall well-being. We are all aware that life gets uncontrollable when stress to take over since it can damage an individual emotionally as well as psychologically. This makes it difficult to continue with your routine activities as you once did, because you're likely to lose your motivation in life. The book's goal is to inspire you, because the bulk of it is making people aware of the power you have to overcome the stress and other challenges in your life. I hope that it can provide you with the information you need to positively influence your life and that of the people in your life.

The first step to healing is to understand the nature of stress it's causes, the symptoms and the effect it could affect your life. It will allow you to be exposed to the truth of it, and, most importantly, educate you on the most effective approach to manage stress and all its manifestations. Nobody deserves to live their lives anxious, and you'll are not just compromising your happiness but also that of your family members. There are many ways to get rid of stressful thoughts and emotions. This book was written specifically for those who be feeling stressed and require effective ways to cope with stress.

It can be difficult to believe in initial stages, however when you begin your journey, you realize that when they open themselves by showing a dedication and willingness, all else will flow in its own way. Tips and strategies for getting rid of stress are fundamental ideas that are able to be integrated into your routine. The majority of them focus on changing your mindset about, emotions and attitude towards things, factors that can significantly contribute to stress levels. The whole process of healing is getting rid of negative energy and becoming open-minded. These are things that a lot people overlook without realizing the significant importance they play in our overall happiness.

The information in this book will not completely eliminate issues and obstacles that you face however, they will show you how to effectively and safely overcome these challenges. It's about looking at the world from a different angle and not allowing any cause be the sole reason to make you unhappy. All your fears, worries anxiety, regrets and worries originate from your mind, and that is why it is important for you to teach your brain to have more positivity. This can only be achieved if you're the one in control, and not letting the mind control you. If it's peace and happiness that you desire that is, then peace and joy you'll receive. All you need to do is allow this book to be your guide throughout that journey every chapter is packed with valuable details. All of it is to help you develop efficient stress management techniques by which you will end up feeling healthier, happier and more effective in your work and personal life.

Chapter 1: What is Stress Management?

If you are aware of the causes of stress but you need to know the effects it has on you, to understand how important it is to manage it. Stress can affect the body and mind and in ways positive and negative. When you are under a lot of stress get sick and exhausted and have a difficult time focusing. difficult to concentrate. It is not uncommon for people to experience emotional and nervous breakdowns. There are two kinds of stress, including positive stress as well as bad. Being aware of these types can help to manage stress better.
Both good and bad
If stress is a problem that is severe enough to lead to illness, then how can be healthy stress? The answer lies in that healthy stress is found in small amounts that increase your physical and mental energy and capabilities to help manage the

upcoming challenges more efficiently and effectively than you would otherwise.

Here are a few examples of stress that are good:

* The stress that is typical prior to an interview for a job or a presentation
* The tension you feel before starting an exercise

In the situations above your energy levels in your body are elevated naturally, increasing your capacity to cope with coming events with ease.

Long-term stress and constant stress are harmful for your body. Your body's tissues will degrade due to the constant pressure of producing chemical substances to manage the stress. Additionally, the an accumulation of these reactions within your body's system as a result due to the absence of a proper outlet externally could increase your stress-related negative side effects.

You are constantly worried about your job
* Stressing over things you cannot control
* Stressing over a loved person's death

In these situations the energy levels of your body do not go up naturally. Indeed, constant stress reduces your energy levels, making you feel tired and unprepared to deal with the challenges of daily life, causing greater stress than ever before. It's an endless cycle that when you are caught up within it, it is extremely difficult to get out from.

What's Stress Management?

The process of stress management is that manages your levels of stress in a balanced and efficient way. The process of managing stress involves identifying the stress triggers, becoming conscious of them, avoiding them whenever possible, and addressing those that are inevitable. Stress management includes a variety of relaxation techniques like meditation or hobbies as well as other activities that can help lower stress levels. What are the benefits of managing stress? It is crucial to manage stress to ensure that stress doesn't become an ongoing issue throughout your life. Stress can cause many problems that include:

* Headaches
* Migraines
* Insomnia
* Weight gain
* Depression
* Digestive problems

Stress management requires acquiring essential skills and understanding to be able to recognize and understand circumstances that can cause stress within your life. With this knowledge and skills, you will be able to find ways to solve the problem and strategies to avoid the triggers or stress that comes from them to the level that is manageable. Stress management is also about developing a plan of action that reduces stress.

There is no one-solution-fits-all option to stress management. Every person is unique, and their reactions and actions are individual. So, it's best to select a method that best suits your needs. Here are some commonly used and fundamental stress management strategies that are applicable to a range of situations and conditions:

Time Management - A lack of time in the form of unlimited time to squeeze into our daily activities is among the most significant sources of stress. There is too much on the plate and there's not much time for relaxation and there is a lot of time spent on unnecessary tasks and other pressures are the result of having an unproductive time management strategy. Effective prioritizing and time management skills are essential for managing stress that you experience in your daily life.

Self-awareness - Being aware your strengths, your ideal levels of energy as well as being aware of when you are pushing your limits and when you are not are all crucial elements that require self-awareness. What's an overly busy timetable for one person might be a breeze for another. The particularity of the techniques for managing stress is what makes them unique. In order for any method to be efficient, you need to first recognize your own limitations . Then, apply the strategies in your own unique area of exercise.

Healthy Diet - A diet that provides wholesome nutrition assists your mind and body to function effectively and allows you to tackle every day challenges with ease. If adequate nutrition is accessible to the body's system, it is less likely to be a problem throughout your day-to-day activities.

Fitness - A regular physical program helps the body shed the stress hormones that accumulate, resulting in decreased stress. Regular exercise routines aid in relaxation of muscles and enhance overall health and health , which can help you to be focused and handle your life's obligations without feeling overwhelmed.

A team of supportive family and friends - taking assistance from loved ones when you are going through a difficult time is among the most effective methods to reduce stress. Being aware that you're not alone to face challenges naturally reduces anxiety as your brain will feel more at ease. Support and encouragement from family and friends is an effective stress-buster. They helped you feel an assurance of security and confidence that can help you handle difficult situations more efficiently.

A good amount of sleep Sleep-related insomnia is a frequent issue that is affecting the world of in the present. In the night, snoring about what might happen or not occur the next morning leaves you exhausted and with no energy to get awake, much less tackle the pressures of the new day.

Sleep is an extremely important component of our lives. The sleep you get lets your mind and body to recover, replenish and refuel to be ready for the the challenges of the coming day. A good night's sleep will keep your body in shape and your mind sharp. In addition your immune system gains strength when you sleep.

It is vital to fall asleep at a specific time each day and make sure you get the rest you need in the evening. This routine can go a ways to reduce stress levels in your life.

The above mentioned elements are some of the most fundamental forms of stress management which all of us need to be aware regardless of professional or social status. Certain of them are covered in greater specific detail in other chapters within the context of this specific situation.

Chapter 2: Define Success

"Success is not the only way to happiness. Happiness is the most important factor to success. If you are passionate about your work, you'll be successful." Albert Schweitzer

Success is greater than our material possessions. It is a concept that can only be defined by themselves. It's that intangible thing that has caused more confusion about this topic than any other. The world has a phobia of intangibles, and is more prone to provide clear examples. So with nothing more precise to go on they have shown the accumulation of power or wealth as the best representation of success. Business executives with a lot of money, powerful politicians and famous personalities are the ones that are most likely to be portrayed as examples in our increasingly distorted society. While power and wealth are considered desirable, it is important to realize that they are not the only elements to be evaluated. The failure to broaden the definition results in a deformed society where we fail to recognize the crucial services provided by people like artists, nurses social workers, etc. who's valuable contribution often isn't recognized. A society in which those who carry out the millions of everyday jobs that keep our society running are not valued or are even viewed as "losers".

We are so fascinated by these false notions of the definition of success, that we give them to our children, as we push them to go into lucrative careers without regards to their actual abilities or passions might be. According to the latest estimates, over fifty percent of Americans are unhappy with their job, and but instead of teaching our children to identify their passions, we keep propagating the notion that wealth accumulation is the only way to success.

The general consensus appears to be that we should be hard-working, which leads to success, which in turn leads to happiness. As psychologists and scientists study the subject in more depth, we are starting to realize that the consensus of the day is interpreting the equation in the wrong way round and that those who deliberately take a path towards happiness tend to be more productive and achieve greater success in the process.

This is not meant to encourage the idea that wealth is always negative and that it is to be celebrated as alternative. The notion is that we pick our own personal version of what constitutes success for us instead of taking the model that the majority of the contemporary world is propagating. Success is an individual thing, and it must remain so for us to realize our full potential instead of settling for an all-inclusive path to success.

One of the dictionary definitions of success includes the accomplishment of a goal or objective. It's a brief definition that is a bit overstates the magnitude of the task. The ability to achieve an objective or goal is one thing, but how do you know if you're uncertain of what your goal or objective should be. A lot of us do not wrestle with this issue and instead believe that the striving for material gains or recognition from our peers is what success about. Do you think it is any surprise that a lot of us feel unhappy at our jobs, don't feel fulfilled or have a nagging feeling of being in failure when these goals aren't attained?

Every person has to define our own standards for success and then take it seriously. In the path to success this could be the toughest hurdle to conquer. It takes time and thorough examination of what our personal values and wants are. As your life changes, your values and desires may change as well. It's likely that you'll need to conduct an extensive assessment of where you are moving at different phases of your life. Your notion of what success means after leaving college might alter when you have kids or your decision is to take a break. Changes like these shouldn't be worried about as long as you are honest about them and don't let yourself be influenced by the dominant opinions of the world around your personal situation or what other people might think about your choice. It doesn't matter whether your vision that you create to achieve your personal goals is that of an successful businessperson or a creative artist. What is important is that you create an image of yourself as successful, regardless of the area of work you decide to pursue. In many ways, these will be among the most crucial decisions in your life. While the remainder of this guide will help you to make these decisions but the final definition of what you consider to be success will be determined by the person you are.

The secret to success in any venture or project is to imagine yourself in the same position at the beginning, and after that you've got something concrete to strive towards. Keep track of the thoughts that go through your head throughout the day. Are these thoughts about achievement and happiness, and staying positive or do they focus on disappointing and failure, and unhappiness? Your attitude can be the main determinant between getting success or ending into a blaze of fire.

Always be aware that the physical world is the reflection of what's happening in your mind world. If all you are thinking about is gloom, doom and failure , then there is no way for you to outwardly show anything else than that.

The more positive and positive your mental images and thoughtsare, the greater chance your physical environment will display positive emotions and attract positive energy.

Your emotions and thoughts are the lenses that you use to see the world, and the way you perceive certain events. The thoughts and emotions you have are also the gauge that your feelings towards the situation are measured. They affect your behavior and reactions. If you constantly visualize and imagine the negative and unhappy and sadness, you won't be capable of seeing the silver linings in any situation , and your actions do not support the silver lining but rather an outcome that is the most negative.

Everyone is unique in terms of emotions, thought patterns and behaviors and each person is focused on different ideas. This is why nobody's response to certain events or circumstances is ever an exact mirror image of another. Someone may have self-consciousness and feel that they don't deserve of being recognized, and this could make them reflect these thoughts and not give the recognition to someone else who might merit recognition. When they do this, they're creating a negative environment that is focused on the things they believe are their own flaws. Someone else may recognize that they have faults, but instead of focusing on their flaws, they will concentrate on their positive and powerful strengths and be perceived as confidence. It allows the person to feel secure. They might be confident enough to share their achievements to others who deserve it. If you are able to emulate the good qualities of these individuals You are sure to get recognition of your own.

A creative visualization is method where you concentrate all of your thoughts and focus on the positive outcome to an event or circumstance and visualize that incident or circumstance positively. The process of picturing success and happiness can draw these things closer. Everyone is able to make use of creative visualization. We are not aware of it. we're doing it without thinking about it and thus not paying attention and using this in a constructive way.

Your mind can be your most trusted friend or adversary. You can train your mind and your self to achieve that goal of achievement and happiness. Be aware of the power within you to achieve your goals. You must stop thinking negative thoughts. Negativity breeds for negative thoughts.

You have to display certain qualities and put them into practice on a daily basis to be able to attain satisfaction and satisfaction. First, you must be confident in yourself and your capabilities. If you are confident in yourself, you provide others reasons to believe as well. In any kind of process. We must be aware that the things that are worth it are not a quick fix and require a lot of effort, so stay patient and you'll reach your goals. Perseverance is a remarkable characteristic that shows your ability to get over your mistakes and doubts and try a new chance. It is impossible to achieve success If you give up after failing a few times. Concentration and determination go together. In the beginning, it's going to require an enormous amount of concentration and mental energy to concentrate your thoughts in a positive way. It is necessary to educate yourself and your mind to be able to process thoughts in a certain waythat you are not used to. You'll need the power of your determination to keep your mind from slipping back into the routines and patterns of thought which have created negative emotions over time. Make it a point to bring yourself to positive thoughts and enthusiasm in the event that your mind begins to drift towards darkness. Self-discipline may be the most difficult thing to attain. To be successful in anything it is necessary to have the drive and ambition to attain your goals. If you are driven, you'll be ready to take whatever steps necessary to reach the place you'd like to be.

It is important to remember that success isn't just is the result of what we do, but also what we are doing. The process of carrying out tasks is crucial, but also the mindset that we are in when doing it. Being able to do the work is essential, but it's not the only thing to consider in this process. Sometimes, we get so caught in the end goals we're striving to reach that we lose sight of the satisfaction that our work ought to bring us. If there isn't any enjoyment or satisfaction while performing the job The task isn't worth the effort. It will become boring and monotonous and you won't focus on it as much. The result or outcome will the process will be influenced.

Get rid of the practices that put the mind in a negative state of mind. Instead, adopt behaviors that encourage your happiness, positivity and happiness that you'd like to experience. Find your unique capabilities and talents, and then pursue your passions and interests. an interest in. Don't try to alter the person you are in order in order to please others or gain the approval of other people. Be content with the choices you make as there is just you as the sole person that has to make these choices.

Be honest with yourself, follow your own personal code of conduct and be brave enough to express your opinions and ideas. Be sure of your value and people will do the same. Confidence radiating from within lets people to feel your confidence and begin to believe in your beliefs and thoughts and get their support behind you.

Believe that success is already within your reach because you are the seed of what the end result will be. You have the power, it's just a matter of learning how to make use of it. You are in control of your future happiness, success and happiness.

Chapter 3: The Two Extremes Of Stress

What do you think are The Two Extremes of Stress?

When it comes to dealing with stress you have two options you should take into consideration. There is the stress-inducing side and the stress-control extreme. This is crucial since there is a solution for the stress you're currently experiencing.

The stress-inducing extreme is situations that cause stress within your life. These are the everyday circumstances that I will cover within this section. Activities that fall within the stress-inducing extremity include:

* Moving into a new home
* Getting into financial troubles
* Going through divorce

Another extreme would be the stress management extreme. It covers the various steps you can take to reduce and removing the stress you feel from a particular situation. The methods you use to control stress may differ in addressing your stress at work.

The extreme of stress management includes the many methods you can employ to stop the effects of stress at work from affecting your home. In this section we will concentrate on the stress-inducing aspect. I will show you how these scenarios can cause stress in your daily life.

Everyday Events That Cause Stress in the Life

Recognizing the triggers that cause stress in a regular basis is vital in managing stress. These are the kinds of events you will experience every day, or at the very least during your lifetime for example, being caught in traffic. These are just a few examples of events which you can easily connect to:

Fighting with your loved Ones or friends

The argument I am referring to in this context is a heated debate which you engage in with a person you don't know. This dispute leads you to say something which you are unable to change which can result in the ending in the relationships. This can be a stressful moment within your life.

After the incident it is common to have emotions of anger and frustration and frustration, accompanied by the realization that you have stopped communicating with a person close to you. The person you cut off communication with was at one time a trusted friend or confidant and the loss of this person can leave a gap within your soul.

Going through A Divorce

Divorce is among the most significant events that cause anxiety throughout our life. Stress remains regardless of an agreement among the spouses. Although you might be happy being free of your ex-partner however, there are pitfalls to this method.

This is due to a few of the steps you have to take in order to finish the divorce. The steps you must take involve court proceedings and addressing the issue about child custody establishing financial arrangements, and the arrangement of your living space. These are just a few of the steps that can cause divorce to be extremely stressful.

The divorce process can have adverse impacts on your children. It's easy to overlook this issue when you are trying to get divorced since the main focus is concerned with your mental and emotional wellbeing. For a child, the separation of parents is often interpreted as because of something they may have done.

Children's inability to express their feelings effectively can make it difficult for them to express themselves. Even with these negative effects however, there are instances where divorce becomes the best alternative. These are the instances when you need to come up with strategies to manage anxiety.

Start by making sure that you have an effective assistance system. The support system isn't just to benefit you but also beneficial for the wellbeing that your kids. It helps reduce the stress your children experience it is essential to keep in touch with your ex-partner, no fighting or arguments with your children.

Staying fit by staying active and physically active can aid in relieving the stress and anxiety that you encounter. In the end, it is crucial to spend time thinking about any decision you choose to make. The emotional turmoil you go through during a divorce could hinder the ability of you to take best choices.

Marriage

Although going through a divorce might appear like something that will never occur in your life however, it is possible for marriage to occur in the near future. This is especially true for someone who's still living a single life. There are lots of things that will change once you make the decision to marry.

Do not get carried away by the joy that comes at a wedding, there are other elements you should think about. Wedding planning is among the many things that cause a lot anxiety. You must find the venue, mail out invitations, and have the wedding gown or dress made.

Also, there is the issue of conflict in the family. How do you convince everyone to be cooperative? What are the steps you must do to make sure everyone is having a blast at the wedding?

Communication is a great option for an enjoyable wedding. Make sure everyone knows what you are planning and how you would like the wedding to run. The next thing to consider is following the wedding.

This is the time begin to adjust to living alongside your loved one. For certain people, they already know what they can expect from their experiences while dating. Some people do not get the chance to experience this. Certain of the experiences you have during your marriage might surprise you.

One of the problems I faced in the beginning in my relationship was related to financial issues. Although I was proficient in adherence to a budget however, I was always having trouble convincing my spouse to follow the same.

This was the main problem in the moment.

The process of overcoming this issue required patience and good communication. In a relationship, communication is crucial. Communicate with your spouse about the things that are causing you pain. This gives you the chance for both of you to come up with a long-lasting solution.

Financial Setbacks

Another life-changing issue that can cause stress is financial difficulties. Insufficient funds to pay your bills, or inability to afford your children tuition fees, and many additional issues that result from the lack of funds could be detrimental to you. This can cause you to worry about the best way to deal with the problem.

There are many reasons you might be experiencing financial difficulties. An investment mistake could play a major role in financial difficulties. If you choose to put your money into an enterprise without doing the thorough research, you could lose all of your investment.

Another reason is your unsatisfactory spending habits. Are you constantly falling into your urges? Are you spending money on things you don't really need? These are spending habits that are commonplace which put you in a difficult spot financially. If you're constantly changing your vehicle or changing from a smaller home to a bigger one is also an issue. This could be a major issue if you're taking credit for these types of purchases. The dependence on credit cards may contribute to financial difficulties.

There are actions you can take to keep yourself from getting into circumstances that can cause stress. They include:

Identifying Your Stressor

Everybody has a stressor, and it might not be the same for others. Recognizing the stressor will be the first step towards solving their financial issues. Some people are often faced with the monthly costs that are greater than their income per month.

Some people are prone to spending habits that lead them to overspend on the credit card they have. To determine your individuality that causes this issue, then you need to look at your spending habits from the viewpoint as an outsider.

If you are able to identify the causes, you have develop a plan to address these issues. If you're prone to impulse buying be sure to restrict the amount of money that you spend when shopping. If the issue is your credit card usage you should consider switching to a cash-only option.

Seek Help if Necessary

The notion that you can overcome your challenges with the help of others is usually the reason you get caught up in difficult situations. Be able to count on others to get through your financial issues. There are probably a lot of acquaintances who know more about managing money than you do.

You may also consult experts for help. In some businesses they have financial health programs that are in place to help employees. If your company has one of these programs, do not be ashamed to join. The thought of what other people will think doesn't offer the solution to your issue. It is possible to lose a number of your friends if they start to consider you a financial risk. Budgeting, debt management and healthy spending habits are a few areas in which experts can help you.

Find Opportunities to Earn More

A little extra money can ease the stress and burden of your financial woes. If you've got a lot of time to spare and are looking for extra jobs to help you meet your financial obligations. The idea of having multiple income streams is also beneficial.

If you are looking to create multiple streams of income it is only possible once you've achieved financial stability. It is important to conduct extensive study prior to beginning this process. This will help ensure you don't get caught in financial problems.

You will discover in the future it is beneficial to reduce your clutter when it comes to earning an extra income. Go through your home looking for items you don't need anymore. Sell them and make money from them. Another car or TV you no longer require can bring you some decent cash.

Not having a job

An occupation is usually one of the most essential things you'll need when you reach the age of adulthood. That is, unless you are an entrepreneur, which allows you to become your own boss. You require a job in order to earn money, and having a career is often a love that drives a lot of people.

Being laid off and having to stay home could cause depression, stress and even humiliation. Stress can be felt when you are worried about making enough money to live on. This is also a problem when you need to change your lifestyle.

Being fired is an immediate strike against your confidence. This is not only having to makes you to discover how to survive on less money. Your situation could be more favorable than the rest if you're intelligent enough to increase your savings even while working.

If you aren't able to quickly adapt to a new way of life There is no way to ease this anxiety. The other option could be find a new job, however, this might not go at the speed you desire it to. This could add to your anxiety when you start to believe that you're not good enough.

While this is understandable it can also be a source of anxiety when you begin an entirely new job. It is possible to quit your current job to take on a new one. What is supposed to be a good thing to be a stressor?

The reason is because new jobs can be difficult. Understanding what your job in the new workplace and creating your new routine have adverse consequences. It's a completely new environment, and you're thinking that you must make an impression.

To lessen the stress of this scenario, the first step is to take a moment as well as ask questions. Engaging with other people can assist you in getting an understanding of what is expected from you. Nobody expects you to know everything about the business on your first day.

They expect that you be able to communicate with other people for help when you require it. This is more effective than doing all by yourself without a partner and making mistakes.

Health Challenges

Another stressor that is common in our lives is health problems. This one can have profound effects on you and the other members of your family. Everyone must make the time to ensure that they're there to support you. This could be physically, emotionally, as well as financially.

There is no need to be hospitalized to be suffering from health issues. This is the reason why it is challenging for people. It is possible that you are experiencing stress in different areas of your life as you are fighting the stress and pain associated with the health issues you face.

The financial burden associated with dealing with health problems could also cause financial difficulties. Certain people are fortunate that they have health insurance coverage that will meet their requirements. Are you among the smart people?

You might think that you don't require health insurance. My opinion is that this is the biggest lie that you can ever tell yourself. It's better to have one but not use it, than to require it but not own it. Life is full of unexpected events.

Injury also falls into this category. The result of accidents, injuries sustained during sporting activities, or accidents that occur at home can cause stress. Imagine being on a wheel chair over the course of the next couple of months. It changes your routine and causes unnecessary stress.

Another issue associated with health problems is that they create unhealthy circumstances. There are people who take up smoking or drinking to alleviate the pain of illness, and to combat depression. When it comes to issues like this self-medication is a different route individuals take.

These aren't the most effective solution. What you must do is to learn more about the situation. Find out about different treatments or consult a physician to seek professional advice as well as take part in support group. If you're able, complete exercises and make sure you're sleeping enough.

They don't make pain disappear in a flash however, they aid in managing your injuries or illnesses. Spend time with friends and participate in activities that bring you joy.

Loss of a loved one close to You

Many people are near to you throughout your life. These are people that have an influence on the way your day runs. What happens if you lose these people?

This isn't a discussion about cutting off communications with a person because of their destructive behavior. What do you deal with the loss of loved ones? It is an event which causes stress and we have no control over these situations.

While we are all aware that death is a fundamental element the human experience, dying can affect all of us in different ways. It could be the passing of parents, spouses an acquaintance, the death of a child. It can be a major disruption to our lives and can cause indescribable sadness.

Certain people might express their sadness in a way of sadness, others as guilt, and others might use anger. This is due to the fact that we don't have a idea how we'll get through our lives without these people. It's an experience you'll need to face sooner or later.

The process of healing after this loss can be long and exhausting. The emotions that accompany this loss can be overwhelming. This is the time in life that you'll need the most support you are able to.

This isn't a trip you should undertake on your own. Rely on other people. Let them know about your pain. This is the way to make progress towards healing.

There are those who never ever fully come back from losing the person they love dearly. The loss causes depression, which causes them to experience an ongoing stress that is hard to get rid of. It is essential to find a way to overcome this particular anxiety to be able to get back to your normal life.

It is possible to seek the assistance counsellors who are professionals who can assist you in overcoming this loss. There are numerous support groups to aid in getting over this hurdle. Make sure you get adequate rest and eating well is essential throughout recovery.

Moving locations

It's fun to have new neighbors come in however, this kind of move causes a lot of anxiety. It can result in a major shift in your life. For those who aren't yet in the process of moving to an entirely new home I'll provide an idea of the stresses that come with this transition.

One of the most difficult things is finding the best location to stay. There are many apartments which you must check out prior to making a decision. You want to find an apartment that is clean with the proper amenities, and at the appropriate price.

Another problem is choosing a new school to the children. This can be stressful for you, but also the children. They will have to adjust to their new school and meet new people.

Finding a home that is easy to get to the bus station as well as one in close proximity to stores and shops is essential. You don't want to have to travel far distances to buy your groceries or replenish products in your store.

If you come up with a solution to deal with these difficulties Be aware that moving into an apartment or a house can put an extra strain on your finances. This is another stressful situation to overcome.

Moving and unpacking your belongings is not a joke. You've probably met the homes of some of your buddies at their new residence and realized that the majority of their possessions are in boxes. Many people find it difficult to break through the mental blockage which is created by the thought of packing.

If you employ someone to help with unpacking or enlist your friends involved to unpack, it can lessen the stress that you are feeling. It is essential to have a support system to help you overcome the emotional strain associated with moving. Chat with your new neighbors, and get involved within the community.

Don't rush to alter your routine when your move is to different place. It takes time to adjust. By doing this slowly, you will reduce the stress you feel.

Your Workplace

A chapter is that is dedicated to our discussion of stress in the workplace. It is among the biggest stressors that affect the lives of many people. This is also that some people experience issues with their home.

Unprofessional management continuous criticism, work hours that is not paid and excessive workloads are a few of the main reasons for stress at work. The effects of this kind of stress can be seen in our relationships with others and in our health.

The ability to manage your time effectively and distribution of your workload could help in the face of stress. We'll discuss more about this in the future.

The Life After Retirement

The lifestyle you will have after retirement isn't easy to plan for. It differs from losing your job in a variety of ways. In one way, you don't have the chance of securing another job.

The transition to a new life can be stressful for a lot of new retirees. It is a shock to realize that, in your pursuit to earn money you did not discover where your most passionate interests are. Your work experience was a factor in your life.

To make it through this drastic change, it takes time. This is essential in altering your routine and coming to be more aware of yourself. This process is more streamlined if have plenty of money in the savings account as well as a 401(k).

Participate in various activities in your community to keep your mind off the problems. Volunteering lets you make use of your knowledge.

Chapter 4: Symptoms Of Stress

Stress is a state of mind that can have consequences for the body, and, in turn, our body affects our psychological state. It is this interconnected characteristics of stress which makes it difficult to comprehend and even more difficult to manage.

Stress is a part of our lives in every aspect. If we're stressed out it can cause psychological, physical or cognitive issues. Here's an overview of ways your body could be trying to inform you of something. You might be surprised by the following:

Physical

Tensions around the neck and shoulders or in the back. Headaches or neck spasms due to involuntarily tightening muscles.

Ulcers, upset stomach or constipation stress can cause our stomach muscles act out in a strange manner.

Changes in appetite or cravings for caffeine and sugar.

Sleep disturbances, nightmares excessive sleep or waking up too early and then being not able to sleep again is a evidence of an active mind.

Weight loss or increase - particularly around the waist due the increased amounts of cortisol.

Low levels of energy.

Emotional

Feeling overwhelmed.

Feelings of sadness, despair or sadness.

A lack of motivation or a desire to pursue what once enthused you.

Repulsion and getting easily annoyed by little things and snapping at people being"short fuse "short fire".

Apathy, self-esteem issues and feelings of apathy

Psychological

Avoiding responsibility and procrastination.

Becoming suspicious, or even fearful of others.

A lack of sexual attraction or desire to see your partner.

Cognitive

The ability to forget things quickly.

Being in "brain fog" and finding it difficult to concentrate on the task in front of you.

It is easy to get distracted.

Finding it difficult to follow things through I'm feeling lost and "all all over all over".

The list above isn't complete. It might surprise you to find out that some people react to stress exactly in the opposite way that you'd think They become depressed and slow, or even depressed.

How we deal with stress can have a lot to depend on our individual makeup as well as our background, whether we're either female or male, our environment that we reside in, and how we've dealt with anxiety in past. Many people experience these signs can trigger the need to take self-medicating drugs like alcohol or drugs and it is a normal response to stress.

Before we get started it is important to be aware of Post Traumatic Stress Disorder, that is a condition that has a level of stress well beyond normal levels. The condition is triggered by a traumatic experience in which the patient was able to feel their life was in danger. The body's reaction could last for months, or years.

If you're suffering from "flashbacks" as well as nightmares about the traumatizing event that occurred to you, and you're constantly stressed or "wired" and are avoiding thinking about or discussing the event it is worth making an appointment with an expert in mental health care to determine if you may suffer from PTSD.

Chapter 5: Develop Long-Term Resilience Habits

Certain techniques for reducing stress If used consistently, could provide the long-term ability to resist stress. This chapter provides the scientific research behind these activities that are most beneficial and provides clear guidelines to adopt these long-term practices. Make use of exercise, meditation, and journaling or a combination of the three.

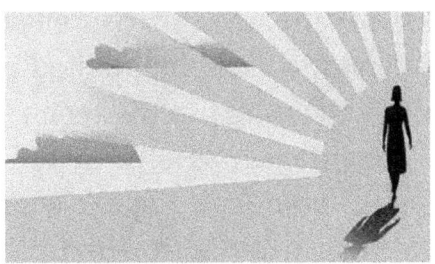

There are many strategies for reducing stress, but not all provide the same degree of flexibility. This chapter offers three efficient strategies to decrease stress. Each one can be learned independently, reap benefits in a matter of minutes, and build benefits over time. Nearly everyone is practicing these. I would encourage you to test each of them and then consider three, two or all three as a part of your daily routine.

Meditation

As you'll recall from the earlier chapter, this effective method has been gaining popularity over the past few years since researchers have found important benefits for reducing stress. Alongside the advantages of meditation in the short term as an effective stress reliever and stress reliever, which I mentioned earlier If you do it in the long run the technique has more advantages. Here are a few advantages you can reap when you meditate consistently for more than a couple of weeks.

There are a variety of meditation that are performed and they all provide benefits in reducing anxiety. Each variation is based on the personal preferences and particularities of various people. Certain forms of meditation are better for one person over others, and certain forms are attractive at various stages of development. The majority of meditation methods can be classified into two major types: centralized and decentralized.

Centralized care strategies concentrate on a specific location. Focusing on the object, feeling or concept is the main focus. This allows for massive shifts in the focus of meditation. The focus point could be an object of light or a mantra or even an item of chocolate, or even the sound of breathing.

Decentralized meditation, also referred to by the name mindfulness, adopts an approach that is more holistic. Instead of paying to an object mindfulness of everything is the primary idea behind this type of meditation: it is stated that the present moment is the primary focus. Focused techniques are easier to master for those who are new however both are equally efficient in managing stress, and both can be applied following the learning process.

Relaxation meditation

The most well-known methods of meditation, especially for those who are new to meditation, is self-meditation. Because breathing is constant smooth, rhythmic and effortless the sounds and the sensations of breathing can be an efficient and efficient method to meditation. Additionally, since meditation operates best with a more relaxed type of breathing, mastering this breathing style and meditative practice tend to complement each other. When our bodies are stressed, the breathing pattern changes to a more shallow and fast pattern. the return to a relaxed rhythm can in reversing the effects of stress and stress, which is why breathing more deeply with meditation to ease stress can be beneficial. In it's own. That's right. Here are the steps to begin a simple breathing exercise:

Find a quiet spot to relax and unwind.

Set the alarm to the time that you would like to work out. (This will let you feel at peace and feel confident that you'll not be unable to complete any important thing to do following the session, or worry about falling asleep , or otherwise awe-inspiring.) To help you adapt to your breathing patterns, you might consider counting every breath, for example taking a breath in two steps, slowly taking 5 inhalations and counting each exhale, slowly, for 8 breaths, while keeping you breathing in a slower rate. It can also provide you with an hour of focus that can help you to get into a more peaceful state, particularly if are just beginning to learn.

You can put aside counting and focus on altering your breathing once you are completely relaxed. Instead of altering your breathing pattern now, you should focus on yourself when you let go of your body. When your mind begins to (and it will) consider other things that your breathing, slowly focus your attention on the sound and feel that your breath produces. You don't need to think about it. Just do it. This is crucial to your training.

You are able to continue the alarm until the sound goes off or you are sure that the session is finished.

This breathing exercise is a basic guideline to help teach and learn, which is a very popular practice for those who are new to meditation. This is among the numerous types of meditation that could be beneficial to you. Here are some of the most well-known kinds of meditation. A brief description of each:

Mantra meditation

This type of meditation can be extremely effective and is easy for those who wish to try other types of meditation. It involves paying attention to a specific mantra, which could be any mantra you wish to use. (Many people prefer to select the sound of om and one that is easy and not compromising to repeat; others prefer words with significance, like peace or hope. Whatever mantra you pick will depend on your own personal preference and you are able to choose according to what resonates with your.) The Mantra Meditation follows the exact method of breathing meditation, apart from repeating the mantra in your head. If you repeat the mantra slowly, when you repeat that phrase (if you do it out loud) you concentrate on the sounds of the word as well as the emotions you experience. While your mind is wandering through other thoughts, gradually return into the mantra.

Musical meditation

The practice of listening to music, in conjunction with meditation, offers substantial advantages. Select music that is soothing and relaxing and concentrate on the music. Let your emotions flow through your body, and then focus on your emotions. Be sure to keep your mind free and focus solely on the sensation.

Meditation on Kindness

The practice, also known by the name of a "goal," can bring positive emotions and thoughts and will help to eliminate the anger and hostility that you may feel towards other people. Instead of being focused upon the phrase, it's an exercise to focus on the feeling of gratitude and love. Be surrounded by positive emotions. Surround yourself with light and love and observe if you feel it inside your body. Think of someone who loves and is surrounded by with love. You can feel it within your body and heart. Go to friends as well as people you do not know, or people who are tired, and then people who are upset or angry. Let all negative emotions that you might be feeling, as that allows you experience positive and loving feelings that take over your thoughts and surround you with the person. It is possible to direct the meditation on kindness to any group of people, and even other nations. Its benefits include reducing anger, depression anxiety and stress and boosting positive social emotions and faith.

Exercise

Exercise is an excellent relief from stress for a variety of reasons. As I mentioned in the previous chapters, physical exercise has numerous benefits, aside from the reduction of stress. These benefits on their own (increased longevity, health and happiness) are enough to make exercising a worthwhile routine. In terms of a stress management method, it's more effective than other methods. The benefits of these two factors are enough to make exercise a daily habit that's worth taking up.

The following kinds of exercise are highly suggested for stress reduction since they possess specific characteristics that help in reducing stress during short and long-term stress management

Yoga

The soft flexibility and balance that yoga provides might be the first thing people think of when they practice, however there are many different aspects of yoga to aid in reducing stress and leading live a healthier life. Yoga is a form of diaphragmatic breathing utilized in meditation. Actually, some styles of yoga include meditation as a part the practice (in fact, all types of yoga will lead you to a certain level in meditation).

Yoga also involves the coordination, balance, stretching and styles. They are all exercises of strength. All are beneficial for the reduction of stress. Yoga can be done in a variety of ways. Some styles of yoga feel like a soft massage on the inside While others sweat and make you feel ill in the following day. So, there's a yoga studio that works for the majority of people, and even those with physical limitations. It is also attractive.

Walking

Walking is among the most efficient ways to alleviate stress , and it is a great choice due to the advantages this approach can bring. The human body was created to move over long distances and the exercise did result in less wear and tear as it does. Walking is a form of exercise that is quickly separated by the speed you are at and the weights you are carrying and the music you play as well as the location and firm you choose.

This kind of workout is also easily divided into 10-minute classes. No special equipment is required and no equipment is required other than the right pair of shoes. (This is a benefit, because studies have proven that three 10-minute sessions provide similar benefits to a 30 minute session. This is a great benefit for people who, due to their busy schedules, require to work out in smaller portions! For more smalls!)

Martial Arts

There are a variety of martial arts and while each might not have a specific emphasis, ideology, or a collection of methods but they all offer benefits to ease stress. These forms of training tend to include the benefits of both strength and aerobic training, in addition to the confidence that comes with self-defense and physical training.

In general, when practiced in groups, martial arts may also provide some benefits of social support because classmates support one another and keep an atmosphere of interaction. There are many styles of martial arts that offer philosophical perspectives that encourage peace and stress reduction and can be a choice to accept or reject. Certain styles, particularly those that involve the highest levels of physical fighting are more prone to the risk of injury. Therefore, the martial arts may not be suitable for all people, or at the very least , not all styles are suitable for every person. If you attempt a few different martial arts classes and consult with your physician before deciding on a type, you'll have an increased chance of finding an exercise routine that will keep your body fit for a long time.

These three examples aren't the only forms of exercise. They are just a few examples of benefits and can be used by a majority of people. There are other types of training that can be highly effective, like Pilates running, exercising with weights dance, swimming and even prepared sports.

Everyone brings their own stress management advantages on the line, therefore find and try the type of exercise that interests you the most.

Journaling

These two methods provide numerous advantages in dealing with stress, and general well-being. While journaling does not bring the same physical benefits as exercise , or provide the same degree of relaxation that meditation does however, it can have positive effects for both mind and body which will increase as time passes. Journaling is also a versatile and easily accessible method, so it's worth a look.

Journaling can trigger certain changes in your emotions (based on the intent behind the practice) and could lead to extreme relief from stress. It can be accomplished in various ways and can take about 5 minutes or even an hour according to the amount of time and goals you might have. If you're not sure you have time to engage in an exercise or meditate in the present you should definitely consider journaling. to think about.

To reduce stress, journaling provides the most extensive benefits that can be expected. It is able to reduce the effects of various ailments, including arthritis, asthma, or chronic pain. It improves the cognitive performance. It strengthens the immune system and can prevent health issues. This could aid in the process of forgiveness. In actual fact, gratitude journaling has been proven to reduce depression over three weeks. Journaling also reduces anxiety.

Based on your preferences depending on your needs, your journaling practices may take any shape you desire. The best option is to create a lengthy note on your PC, which contains articles that relate to your day. Write in a stunning rainbow font, or write your thoughts on a series of articles. Write them on the inside of your. Mirrors in the bathroom or even one or more hosts. Explore different alternatives. (My journaling has used various forms over the years and many more).

However, certain techniques for writing have proven to be effective in achieving certain goals. Here are a few different methods of journaling that appear to have the most effect in reducing stress. Whatever method you use to write your thoughts (digitally or in multicolored ink, or even in steam tracking) These focus areas are a great idea.

Journaling focusing on emotion We all have issues that can cause stress. Examining the stress that we feel and examining the causes of our feelings can help us to transcend anxiety and worry and find a space for peace within.

Journaling with a focus on solutions

The use of journaling techniques to reveal emotions can help us find emotional freedom and deeper roots to our lives. Techniques that focus on finding solutions to stressors may be efficient in aiding the process of releasing stress-inducing emotions. This is especially true when you are feeling anxious or gossip, and steps can be taken to alleviate this.

Gratitude Journaling

Journaling is widely acknowledged and has numerous advantages that are echoed here. Journaling with gratitude will be a significant factor in emotional well-being to the extent that depression can increase.

Journaling that is goal-oriented

Journaling can help the awareness of the environment you reside and which situation you must be. It is possible to identify the goals you want to achieve and then break them down in smaller pieces. After that, you can track the progress you make. This makes it easier so that you can progress through the various levels of change. It will allow you to acknowledge yourself on your accomplishments and allow you to get the maximum amount of distance in your plans. You can also swap your notes. It is an enjoyable and authentic way to journal and doesn't require regular writing.

Beginning to journal

Journaling is easy to maintain, however, as with every newly developed habit there's some things to remember. The habit is not effective in the absence of a regular do it regularly, particularly with gratitude journaling. Note that shorter entries that are regularly written could benefit from longer-length entries that appear to be working. The entries are rarely written. Keep in mind that you can journal anytime and if you've not journaled in your magazine for a while, you can backup it and continue writing. Here are some suggestions to consider before you begin:

Pick your location. As we mentioned there are a variety of options to create your own diary. Many people enjoy the convenience of recording their thoughts on a computer, whereas others appreciate the traditional feel of paper and pencil. Sometimes, a gorgeous diary may inspire you to create more detailed notes and for some it is better to use a book that will reduce the pressure to write pieces with content that is "deeper" than the authentic ones. Consider what is most suitable for you and your preference. Remember that If you're concerned about privacy make sure you protect your privacy. Journaling works best in the absence of having to be censoring yourself.

Pick your style. If you have read the previously written descriptions of journalistic techniques that focus on emotions as well as focused solutions and gratitude It is possible that one particular style appeals to you. It is possible that you will find that different types of journaling are best suited to different scenarios.

If you feel you've felt like you are in a noise and you are struggling to deal with them, you're at a heightened level, even though you're busy. Thank you. You feel sad and unsatisfied and you want to look the best elements of your life. Remember that the journal you want to write about as well as how you wish to feel, as well as the way you journal are easier to decide on.

Be flexible. If they don't like you for a couple of days, don't let them go. If your writing is filthy (or your writing is full of mistakes) It's okay. If you plan to write about three things that you're thankful for, and what you could come up with three, those are two things that will positively impact your life! Do you require taking photos with your writing? Are you able to be relaxed and flexible in your training? This can make the habit simpler and more enjoyable. You should ask yourself questions

What are my goals in managing my stress? Do I need to relieve physical stress, lessen anxiety, ease mild depression, and work on relaxation techniques?

Which one of these options is the most straightforward for me to accomplish?

What advantages can I expect from each of these practices?

What are the ways these ways of living fit into my life?

Can anyone assist me in keeping the track of them?

What other help will I require to live my best life?

(If you've not tried any of these methods in the past , but haven't resisted this routine) When I last attempted to sustain my habit was what stood blocking me? What could be differently this time?

How can I help make an impact?

Assess Your Responses

In order to be able to sustain a long-term dependence, you must commitment. It lets you know exactly what you must accomplish and the reason behind it. The search for answers will allow you to identify the issues that will help you through the process and help you be back on the right path if you are lost.

Knowing what you'd like to achieve will help you make the best decision. If, for instance, you're looking to cleanse your mind of thoughts that cause stress A daily journal addiction will help you organize the thoughts that are in your thoughts. An exercise session can help you clear your mind and alter your perspective and allow you to respond less to anxiety over time. Meditation can achieve the same goal however in a different way which is why understanding your own needs and retaining your goals can be helpful.

If you take a look at your results to the questions, you need to keep them in the mind that you are motivated. You'll be able to see what strategies you'll need to do to stay on track, and what you should do if you fail to follow through. In the next chapter, you'll learn more ways to enforce these responses to your life.

Chapter 6: Habits of Life that ease stress

Smoking or drinking excessively and not getting enough rest drinking too much caffeine, and being around people who make you feel stressed can cause anxiety levels going through the sky. If you're trying to quit these unhealthy habits to reduce anxiety and stress Which ones are most effective to replace them with? In most cases, replacing a habit with another one could be an effective method to aid in the process of quitting the one you started. For instance, people who smoke might choose to switch from smoking cigarettes to vaping, which isn't as hazardous, yet gives them something to do rather than smoking cigarettes. Many prefer to exchange unhealthy habits for ones which are totally different. for instance drinking often may decide to take up exercising to give themselves something to do, instead of taking drinks.

Exercise

There's the entire chapter of this book already to exercise however it's so crucial that it should be mentioned once more. Regular exercise is among the best habits you can adopt for improving your mental health and ensuring you're stress levels remain in control. Participating in sports like cycling, walking, running or swimming, yoga as well as weight-lifting or participating in a team sport can help improve your physical fitness, boost fitness, and increase confidence and self-esteem. All of which will help reduce anxiety and stress. The exercise itself releases positive chemical substances in the brain and has been scientifically proven to help reduce symptoms of depression and anxiety.

Meditation

In the fight against anxiety, meditation is an excellent habit to pick to incorporate into your routine. Since the beginning of time meditation has been used to assist people with anxiety and stress levels and to feel more peaceful in their own skin.

Meditation can help you find the positive energy within you and make you be more connected and at peace with the world around you. Regularly practicing meditation can help you discover that stressful circumstances do not afflict them as they used to. They are more calm at ease, relaxed and capable of taking on increasing amounts of. If you're a spiritual individual or not there's no doubt that mindfulness-based meditation can make you be more relaxed and feel at ease. The act of sitting down in silence and take a moment to take your thoughts in for a bit will help lower stress levels, since the practice requires that you take deep breaths and increase the oxygen levels in your brain and provide you with more energy to manage your anxiety. Mindfulness meditation can be performed at home or in the form of a class. You may also make use of various essential oils and music to help you.

Creativity

The ability to be creative is one of the most effective ways to combat stress. The best part about using your imagination to tackle anxiety is the fact that one doesn't need to be a particularly talented artist to be able to do it successfully. There are many studies that directly link being creative with less stress and stress levels, with adults coloring book and apps to combat stress being extremely popular. The act of coloring with images, or engaging in a creative activity like making cakes, needlework or even DIY, can be therapeutic and allow you to shift your mind and help you focus on your worries and instead focus on other things. So, if you're exhausted, it might be time to consider engaging in a new creative activity.

Friends and Family

Mentally strong people are not able to separate them from the people close to them. If you're stressed it's easy to conceal your anxiety from close family and acquaintances because naturally, it isn't your intention for them be concerned about you. But knowing when to request help and having the right people around you to provide is crucial in successfully managing stress. Establishing and maintaining strong relationships with your close family members and friends can ensure that you have someone to talk to whenever things get difficult that is extremely beneficial for stress. Talking to someone and share your thoughts about what is causing you stress will give an outsider's view and can help in putting your thoughts in a different perspective. In addition having someone to talk to can help stop you from getting too stressed out and give you time to relax and remain up with your mental well-being.

Chapter 7: Considering the Life Cycle

The majority of the written accounts on stress address the subject in a general medical and scientific approach to every person, regardless of the age. A few, or none ever see stress and its causes, symptoms or symptoms, as well as its impact according to the cycle or the stages of life. However, of course the final phase, death, is not included. Stress is impossible for a body that is dead.

There are six phases of the human life cycle: (1) pre-birth or pregnancy; (2) birth/newborn to infancy, or between 0 and 3 years old; (3) childhood or between 4-12 years old; (4) teenage years/adolescence or 13-21 years old; (5) adulthood; and (6) death. By using the lens of gender the male and female humans are believed to have different reactions to body in response to stressors. This is because , according to the latest research, the emotional quotient of females continues to be higher than male. This is the only area of emotional self-control that women fail to achieve higher scores, however there isn't a gender gap. was found in an article written by Lipman in Forbes.com.

Stage 1: Pregnancy or pre-birth. The book I wrote in Positive Parenting Parents What makes you an Exceptional Parent that Children Love is that a child in the womb of a mother is affected by the way that a mother is a food lover and complains about becoming overweight, feeling uncomfortable or aching even experiencing constipation. The child in a mother's womb is able to be influenced by everything that a mother is experiencing, so the human body is subject to stress during the pregnant women. What is the reason?

The stress of pregnancy is regarded as a source of stress to women, which is which is why she can become emotionally. The concern of being overweight as well as the fear and stress in pregnancy are the factors that cause stress for mothers, but not for a baby. It is the sensation of being emotionally stressed that can become the main stressor for children in the womb. The stress of a mother's life is not the same as that of the baby in the womb, but rather the effects of stress on the mother. The nutrients that are present in mother's diet can trigger stress in the event that it affects the health of the baby inside the womb. Any change in the body's system of a mother could cause stress to an infant in the womb.

The effects of stress on children during pregnancy might not be apparent immediately, except for mothers who are drug or alcohol dependent and smoke. Smoking and drinking alcohol can result in birth defects. Stress during pregnancy may impact the baby after birth. This can affect the emotional quotient, behavior or cognitive abilities.

Stage 2: Infanthood or the period between 0 and 3 years old. age. A vulnerable stage of life, where a child begins to master everything, starting with talking or crawling to walking, and recognizing objects that surround the child. If a child does crying indicates that they are experiencing stress. The crying is a normal part of growing older and it's good for your heart. The excessive crying is known as colic. Colic is the term used to describe excessive crying with no reason at all. Although there isn't a medical condition that is currently linked to colic, it's nevertheless a source of stress for the child as well as naturally for the mother or the nanny.

The main causes of stress for an infant at this point is sensitivity to food or milk, not having mother's focus, being around unknowing children around becoming exhausted, losing toys, experiencing pain and suffering from an illness. In accordance with this American Psychological Association (APA) classification of anxiety, baby anxiety may be episodic or acute. Chronic stress can occur in babies who have congenital disorders.

The effects of stress on infants isn't too alarming and is easily managed or rectified. Infants cry when they are hungry or when stomachs are upset due to the milk or food eaten. Giving a child food as well as a dose of medicine could be the answer. A child's cry when their sleeping environment is unsuitable or is not capable of sleeping or sleep, a soothing lullaby from the mother can be effective. The only exception is congenital illnesses.

The 3rd stage is called Childhood, or 4-12 years of age. The time in which the development of a person is beginning to grow and where curiosity is high. A child of this age group is always asking questions. What is more difficult is to respond to all of their endless questions. Mothers everywhere will be able to relate to this. Also, children have a higher proportion of retention of information. Because the learning curve in the early years of childhood is in an increased rate it is not easy to see the effects of stress isn't immediately. Parents and mothers must be aware of. In particular, causing an increase in anxiety that is stressful could affect a child's confidence levels now and in the future. It is worth noting that the stress of children's emotions is usually deeply rooted.

At this point when the triggers of stress began to rise. The reason for this is that the involvement or influence of outside actors increase or a child starts to engage with others externally. Alongside siblings, children begin relationships with classmates, relatives and friends, neighbors or not. The main reasons for sibling stress include petty disputes and rivalries with parental attention as well as toys and bullying. Apart from the attention of parents The same can be the most common reasons for stress in your schoolmates and neighbors. The stress of schoolwork is more a case of episodic stress.

Children are innocent and innocent Stress isn't that dangerous to a child , unless there is the stress of divorce and death, which could have a lasting effects on children's development. Parents' comfort is the best method of managing stress up to the point of no return. Doctors and medicine are secondarily to congenital illnesses, unless they are congenital.

Stage 4: Adolescence/Teenage Years which is 13-21 years old. This is the time when the possibility of suicide is present and other untoward behaviors could occur if they are not addressed or arrested at an early point. The causes of stress at this stage were mostly derived from external factors like classmates, friends at school as well as relationships, school performance and. Family and the relatives not the main source of stress. This is also the time when teenagers begin to recognize family problems and financial struggles. They are aware of the reasons of divorce between parents.

Teenagers put an emphasis on the integrity of their lives and giving a good impression is paramount. A teenager who is afflicted with anxiety is likely to avoid. However, the effects of the stress caused by humiliation may last for a long time, and could even lead to death. Physical appearance and characteristics can be another source of stress and could influence teens' confidence levels. Funny how a pimple on the face can make you feel anxious at times.

Because this stage is vulnerable to stress that is chronic and could be fatal, the necessity to seek medical interventions was first identified. Medical and counseling are recommended to prevent unintentional behaviors and to avoid the onset of depression in a certain degree. Stress can last for a long period of period if not addressed or stopped at an beginning. Other signs of that stress can trigger are an inability to connect with social and physical communication, crying eating too much or not eating, sleeping too much and skipping classes.

Stage 5 Stage 5: Adulthood. The extensive list of stress-related causes and the variety of symptoms that can be observed at this point. It is at the stage of adulthood that the highest level of stress can be discovered. Stress that is acute can lead to illness and a variety of symptoms, while chronic stress can trigger Depression and even suicide. The ability of individuals to deal with stress can vary, based on age, experiences and exposure to stressors.

What differentiates this stage from the previous stage is the ability of an adult to conceal and to handle stress by themselves. This is not self-treatment however, it is the ability for an individual to locate the inner strength required to deal with or alleviate stress. Some find relief through the arts and music. Others refer to it as an enlightenment, when they seek faith and missionaries, and work to treat.

Stage 6 Stage 6: Death. The final phase of the cycle of life is death, when stress doesn't matter anymore. Stress is a burden for the ones who have passed away.

Stress and the Human Life Cycle

There are six phases of the human experience: (1) pre-birth or the pregnancy stage; (2) birth/newborn to infancy, or between 0 and 3 years old; (3) childhood or between 4-12 years old; (4) teenage years/adolescence and 13-21 years old; (5) adulthood; and (6) death.

The mother's stress is not the same as that of an infant in the womb but rather the consequences of stress to the mother. The effects of stress on children during pregnancy might not be evident immediately except for mothers who are alcohol/drug dependent or smokers.

The process of crying is normal for growing children and is beneficial for your heart. Colic or prolonged crying might not have a medical problem connected to it, but prolonged crying caused by stress needs to be taken care of.

The effects of stress on a baby isn't alarming and can be easily controlled or remedied. Stress can be chronic in babies who have congenital illnesses.

The child's first interactions are with their siblings, schoolmates, the neighbors or friends, or neither. They are the main source of tension. Parents' comfort is the most effective method for managing stress up to this point. Doctors and medicine are secondarily with respect to congenital disorders.

Adolescence is a stage that is susceptible to stress that lasts for a long time It is during this time that the need for medical interventions began.

It is during the adulthood phase that the highest level of stress is reached. Stress can cause illness and a variety of symptoms, while chronic stress can cause Depression and even suicide. The capacity of an individual to manage stress can vary, depending on age, experiences and exposure to stressors.

Chapter 8: Quick Tips To Manage Stress

The advice included in the chapter could be applied immediately if you start to notice the warning signs! These are short-term strategies that are efficient in relieving anxiety. You can adjust them depending on your own personal preference that best suits you.

Breathe into the paper bag, then breathe.

It may sound straightforward however, trust me in this case. It is possible to take an empty bag of paper and begin breaths into it while you breathe. Utilize this technique either prior to stress or even during tension.

What can it do for you? It regulates the way you breathe and allows you to concentrate on one task at a time. In time, your breathing will resume normal and the sense of being secure would begin to be felt. Then, you will feel more comfortable and take care of the issue at hand.

Get away from the situation

You can hold or move off from your situation if it begins to cause stress. Go for a walk, or leave to go to the bathroom or make a fake phone call you have to make.

When you do this you are giving yourself some time to breathe and allow yourself time to think about the situation. Do not let it become an overpowering level! Make an effort to deal with it in the time that you have.

Depressing activity

Once the stress begins to set in, close your eyes take a deep breathe and begin counting your fingers as you rub your palms gently as you try to picture your clothing all the way down and then try to recall your thoughts as you close the eyes gradually. Remind yourself by telling yourself, "It is going to be okay, just breathe in, breathe."

The activity diverts your attention from stress and relaxes your mind. By using your fingers to count as you rub your palms while visualizing the process, you convey the feeling of safety to your body. This will help reduce stress levels.

Perform these easy tasks

Follow these easy steps to lower your stress levels.

Drink water

Play your favorite song.

Use a gum chew to relax your jaw

Take a whiff of your favorite scent. (Citrus scents work best for decreasing anxiety levels.)

Watch a fun video

Make sure you light your candle of choice

Get some flowers

Let it go

It can be overwhelming when the stress cycle starts and you begin to think about, analyze and overthink every single detail. When you let things go you develop a new perception of the situation and the sense of fear diminishes. It is also clear how hazy the thought process was and how nothing could ever be happening. Therefore, choose one of the methods mentioned to relieve tension.

Talk with yourself and talk about the current situation.

Speak to a trusted acquaintance and ask for help.

Note it down as you feel and then release it.

Have a shower or bath.

If you are able to get a shower, or take a bath, I suggest you to do it. Your muscles become more tense during stress, so having a bath can relax you and ease tension. Make use of your preferred soap or shower gel, or Body butters, light a few candles, turn on your preferred music and take a moment to appreciate how lucky you are in this particular moment. Take a moment to unwind and reflect on the amazing things, things you're grateful for.

Try laughter therapy

The therapy of laughter is simple and will give you the best results. When you smile, your body immediately releases the hormones that make you feel good (endorphins) that aid in reducing stress. If you're anxious and lonely, push yourself to be as loud that you are able to. If you're in need of inspiration and a laugh, try laughing in a strange way or mimic the laugh of someone else. If you're not able to make a loud, loud laugh, smiling can help produce endorphins.

Take care to get things in order

Unorganized spaces, clutter, and changes can cause stress. If you see the appearance of clutter, chaos around the house or changes you do not like take a step forward and put things organized. Be wary of feeling lazy or shy and do whatever you have to do to feel better.

Shut down your account

Social media is the main source of stress. People not responding to your messages, looking at your life in comparison to others and being constantly available to you 24 hours a day and the constant need to impress people all the time of your day can be stress-inducing. When stress begins to take over take a break from all social media platforms Be quiet, relax your body. Stay clear of any social media interaction you don't feel at ease with until you are at ease.

Do the most drastic thing

If you are experiencing stress caused by abuse, bullying or harassment, you should take legal action or notify the authorities. Don't take it on in a quiet way and don't confront the issue on your own. Make sure you are able to take the first and last step toward your abusive partners. If you are unsure of whether you're not able to make a report, talk to a reliable person, such as a general physician or guidance counsellor, or an organization for support. Ask for assistance.

Sing an original song

You may be amazed at how singing can ease tension and allow you to feel lighter! A good singer, a not-so-good singer, just sing! in the privacy of your own home as you go for on the walk, or as you jam to your iPod. Find a track you love, or even make your own. Try it and you may notice that your day getting a bit more cheerful.

Have a massage

Massages are the most relaxing thing can be attempted to relax your body and mind. Massages make you feel relaxed and rejuvenated. It eases tensions and knots of muscles. Massages are often helpful in releasing emotional tension (stress) within the body. It is recommended at least scheduling massage every once each week, particularly in case you're feeling stressed, it will make an immense impact.

Take a dip in the sunshine

Vitamin D aids the body reduce stress. If you suffer from an insufficient amount of vitamin D it will cause higher amounts of stress. Sunlight is a great supply of Vitamin D. Set a routine to lie in the sun for about 10 minutes throughout the daytime. Being in the sun improves your mood and helps you feel healthier.

Remind you

Keep a positive attitude and conviction that things will improve. Maintain your self-confidence and faith in the highest level because it will assist you through difficult moments. Keep a record of the memories you have made through difficult times in your life. You can then analyze how you handled the challenges. Be confident in yourself and don't quit.

Zoom out of your life

Stress can arise when we are thinking too highly of ourselves and believe that everything is in our control. Stress is a natural reaction when we think the issue is more significant than it is and keep in analyzing it. Try to take a look at the larger view that you live. Don't get caught up in the little issues! Many of the things that make us scream do not really matter at all. Take control of the things you can manage. This way, you'll be able to be able to see the bigger picture and it doesn't seem as daunting.

Buy/adopt a pet

If you're experiencing anxiety or stress levels that are high you should consider buying or adopting pets! With endless cuddles, affection, companionship and support, many people have seen a dramatic decrease in their anxiety levels following the introduction of pets into their lives.

Be surrounded by the beauty of nature

Nature soothes the mind and soul. mind. If you're feeling exhausted, take a long cycle or walk through the woods, the mountain trails, or a picturesque park, and be awed by the natural world. Enjoy the beautiful scenery of the environment you live in! It is also possible to incorporate plants within your workspace or home perhaps you're interested in trying gardening.

These are a few simple strategies that can be extremely efficient in dealing with anxiety, right in the moment. Which one of these is most compatible to your lifestyle? What are some new things that you might explore?

Chapter 9: Relaxation Techniques

We've already discussed ways to reduce stress, so it's time to talk about the best methods to reduce stress. Relaxing is the most effective way to ease stress, but you must know how to relax in a safe and healthy way. Here are some suggestions to ease stress and relax. stress in healthy and productive methods.

Speak to someone about the issues you're experiencing. Sometimes, just talking with someone about your issue can help you feel better even if they are unable to offer any assistance to the situation. It is comforting to know that someone is willing to listen.

Relax with relaxing music. It can help you relax and allow you enough time to think things over.

Do some taking deep breathes. It can help relax you and increasing the oxygen flow into your brain. It also reduces blood pressure and heart rate. Breathe slowly into your nose, and then out through your mouth.

Make something new and interesting. It could be anything that you love doing such as playing instruments, drawing, or painting. It can help keep your mind away from the stress and let you relax to allow you to think more clearly.

Exercise is among the most effective things you can do to unwind yourself, and also provides many health benefits.

Meditate. A few minutes of meditation can ease stress. Repeating a mantra may help you focus when you meditate.

Slow down. If you feel stressed or overwhelmed, you can slow down. Take a moment to be present. Focus on the things you're doing in the moment. If you're eating, take pleasure in the flavor of the food. Concentrate only on your food.

Take a listen to pop or rock music. If you're feeling stressed or angry Listening to loud music might be just what you need. You are free to sing and move to the beat.

Take an appointment for a massage. A massage can soothe not only your body , but as well your mind.

Hypnosis. Sometimes, other techniques for relaxation don't apply to everyone. If you're looking to think outside of the box, or simply want in seeing what it is like, you should consider the hypnosis method.

Whatever you do to help you relax and is also beneficial to your health is a beneficial way to relax. Explore different options until you discover something that is suitable for your needs. You must make sure you use your relaxation strategies along with positive skills for coping such as positive thinking, problem-solving, along with time management.

Chapter 10: Social Stress

Social stress concerns relationships in general and within the context of other people. According to the notion of evaluation of emotion, the issue occurs when an individual believes that they lack the skills to handle or deal with the situation that is specific and evaluates an event. Because the risk of an incident can be sufficient, an event which is more than the capabilities is not required to trigger anxiety. There are three types of fears. Life events are described as sudden dramatic life altering circumstances that require one to be able to react quickly (ex. Sexual attack, sudden harm). Chronic breeds are defined as events that are persistent and require a person to make changes over a long period of time (ex. Divorce, unemployment). Everyday problems tend to be described as small incidents that occur that require to be addressed throughout your day (ex. horrible congestion (disagreements). That could put you at risk of getting ill as well as physical 29. Stress persists and one experiences mental, behavioral and physical changes? Social beings are by nature. They are driven by the need to stay connected to their social networks and needs. Therefore, they consider keeping positive connections to be advantageous. Social networks are an integral part of achievement and may provide feeling of acceptance. Anything that could cause disruption or can threaten to break their bonds could cause societal Stress. This could include having a low social standing or at certain classes, giving a talk or interviewing potential employers, taking care of the child or partner with an illness or chronic condition and meeting new people at an event, the possibility of death or the loss of a loved one divorce or separation, and even discrimination. Stress in the social sphere can be triggered by both the macro-environment (e.g. relationships with family members) and the macro-environment (e.g. (Hierarchical Social Structure). Social stress is a type of stressors that affect the lives of others more deeply and feel daily.

Definitions Researchers define anxiety and stress in a variety of ways. Wadman, Durkin, and Conti-Ramsden (2011) defined social stress as "the feeling of anxiety or anxiety people confront in social settings and the corresponding tendency to avoid potentially uncomfortable social settings." Ilfield (1977) described the term "social issues" as "conditions that arise from social interactions which are typically regarded as undesirable or unsuitable." Dormann as well as Zapf (2004) defined the social issues as "a class of behaviors or events or behavior that is related to psychological or physical stress, and are socially oriented."

Measurement

Social stress can be quantified using self-report questionnaires. With the help of protocols and various strategies researchers may create Stress in the laboratory.

Self-Reports

There is psychosocial stress. Self-reporting steps for self-report consist of those that include the Evaluation of Negative Social Exchange and The Marital Adjustment Test The Risky Families Questionnaire, the Holmes-Rahe Stress Inventory and the Trier Inventory to assess the severity of Persistent Stress The Daily Stress Inventory as well as the Job Content Questionnaire, the Perceived Stress Scale as well as the Stress and Adversity Inventory. Researchers can use evaluations of interviews. For example, the Life Activities as well as the Life Events Difficulties schedule (LEDS) is one of the most frequently used tools for research. The purpose of this type of steps is to force players to discuss their most stressful life experiences, instead of answering questions that are awe-inspiring. It is the UCLA Life Stress Interview (LSI) which is a lot similar to the LEDs, includes questions on romantic partners and close friendships, as well as other social associations and family relations.

Induction

In rodent-based model, the concept of defeat as well as disruption are two concerns that are commonplace models. Inside a cage rodents are introduced into the chaos paradigm rodents naturally have established the structure of a hierarchy. The aggressive "intruder" interferes with the social structure, creating the residents to feel stressed out. Within the social defeat model an aggressive "intruder" and a different male rodent that is not aggressive fight. In a study on humans there is a Trier Social Stress Task (TSST) is employed to incite Stress. In the TSST participants are told to prepare and present a talk about the reasons they're a good candidate for their position. The participant films while they give the speech and inform the participant that a panel of judges will be evaluating the speech. After the speaking portion an exercise in math that involves counting backwards in increments is conducted by the participant. The researcher will prompt the participant to start if the participant commits a mistake. The possibility of being judged could be your trigger. Researchers can evaluate the stress response through analyzing the levels of salivary cortisol before stress and the levels of salivary cortisol after stress. Other stress-related measures that are commonly used at the TSST include self-reporting steps like the State-Trait Stress Inventory, as well as physiological measures like the heartbeat. Couples are able to identify specific regions of conflict. The couple then pinpoints couple of subjects to discuss later in the course of their experimentation (ex. financing, child-rearing). Couples should review the conflict (s) in a 10-minute period while they are being recorded. Brouwer as well as Hogervorst (2014) developed their Sing-a-Song Stress Evaluation (SSST) create stress in the lab setting. After watching Pictures with backrests, intervals are taught to sing a song complete. Researchers have discovered that the conductance of the skin and heart rate are both higher. Through the time period of the message when compared to previous intervals. The stress levels are comparable to those.

Statistics of Stress Signs In Massive Groups

An analytical stress index Correlations and variance was recommended for the detection of Stress and was used in physiology and finance. The analysis of catastrophes proved its usefulness in identifying areas of a cause of concern in classes. The study was conducted in the aftermath of the stress-related period, which was beyond the political and the 2014 Ukrainian economic disaster. There was a increase in the connection between the 19 most significant public anxieties that exist in Ukraine Ukrainian social structure (roughly 64 per cent) and their dispersion in the statistics (by nearly 29 per cent) during the preceding decades.

Mental Health

Studies have shown that Stress can increase the risk of causing adverse health consequences. One potential study requested more than fifteen hundred Finnish workers whether they had "significant difficulties with [they are] coworkers/superiors/inferiors throughout the past six weeks, five decades, before, or not." Information on hospitalizations, suicides, for suicidal behaviors as well as psychosis, alcohol dependence symptoms, and medications for psychiatric issues were collected from the death registers and morbidity. Individuals who had a conflict in the office over the last five years with their managers or colleagues were more likely to be diagnosed with an illness. The people who have been identified by studies on the LGB population. LGB have mental health issues like alcohol and mood disorders as compared to. Researchers conclude that LGB individuals' risk of developing mental health issues stems from their stressful environment. Minorities are often confronted with significant levels of stigma as well as discrimination and prejudice often, which leads to the development of mental health problems.

Depression

The likelihood of developing depression is higher after experiencing stress. Prior to becoming miserable, people who are depressed often suffer from social loss. One study showed that it was diagnosed with depression three times as fast. In a population, people with relatives and friends who are critical of their requirements and cause tension and conflict, frequently exhibit symptoms. The conflict between spouses can lead to an increase in Psychological anxiety and depression symptoms particularly for wives. In particular, married couples ' 10--25 times more at risk for developing depression. Social stress is linked to greater stomach symptoms. In one research, whites referred discrimination experiences and depression symptoms. No matter what race, those who believed in perceptions had depressive symptoms.

Stress

The biological foundation for stress-related disorders lies in the activation of the stress response. Fear, the most defining emotion in a disorder of stress can occur when a person experiences a situation (a threat) as frightening. The stress response is activated. This can occur if someone is struggling to control this stress response. Stress may occur when something threatens to happen or the exact trigger isn't there. This could result in the creation of a stress disorder (panic attacks or anxiety, social tensions OCD and OCD..). Stress disorder in social settings is defined as the anxiety of being judged or evaluated by others even when no risk exists. Studies have shown a connection between Stress and trauma, like life events and strains and the development of stress-related disorders. A study that examined an adult subset who were young and middle-aged and found that those who were been diagnosed with a disorder of stress during their adulthood were victims of sexual assault. Children who experience issueslike reduction, as well as injuries, are more prone to develop stress-related disorders as in comparison to kids who did not have to deal with stressors through adulthood.

Long-Term Consequences

Social stress can have effects that last or become apparent as you mature. A longitudinal study showed that children were significantly more likely to suffer from an illness of the psyche (e.g. manic, stress personality, as well as alcohol-related disorders) in the latter part of adolescence and early adulthood when parents showed more inadaptive behavior towards children (e.g. the loud argument among parents, abuse verbally and inability to control anger toward the child, insufficient parental care or accessibility as well as painful punishment). Child temperament and psychiatric illnesses have not been able to clarify this relationship. Studies have revealed connection between children and stress with suicide, stress and melancholy depression as well as antisocial behavior, family environment and the environment, as well as aggressive, hostile and disruptive behavior.

Relapse and Recurrence

Stress can worsen psychological disorders and cause a slow the process of recovery.

For instance, people who are recovering from bipolar disorder and depression are more likely to return in the event of tension. Patients suffering from eating disorders tend to suffer more in the event that their family members are violent to make critical remarks or are too involved. The same is true for those with eating disorders. more severe symptoms are observed in patients who are outpatients suffering from schizophrenia or schizoaffective disorders who are in a position where their life is significant and more likely to suffer relapses in the event of Stress affects their relationships.

Concerning chemical abuse, report higher levels of craving for cocaine following exposure to social stressors. Stressful life events and social problems can trigger the deterioration of symptoms of mental health disorders. The condition can become unresponsive and less prone to avoidance.

Physical Well-being

The results of research have revealed a link between different stressors and aspects of health.

Mortality

Social standing, a stressor is a reliable predictor of departure. In a study that included over 1800 British civil service workers and their socioeconomic position (SES) was found to be inversely linked with mortality. The people with the lowest SES suffer from poorer quality of life and mortality rates are higher than those with higher SES. Numerous studies have demonstrated the link among SES and mortality for various diseases, including digestive, infectious and respiratory illnesses. A study that examined the relationship between SES and mortality in the elderly showed that family income and occupation prestige were linked to decreasing mortality in males. For women, however only real household income has been linked with a lower risk of dying.

Similar to this, social stressors from the micro-environment could also contribute to an increase in mortality. An analysis of a seminal longitudinal study of more than 7,000 individuals revealed that those who were socially isolated had an increased risk of dying due to other reason. Social support, which is described as "the support, relaxation and guidance one receives through informal or casual contact with individuals or groups," has been linked to physical health consequences. Research has shown that regular interactions and the three dimensions of perceived social support may predict mortality for thirty months later.

Morbidity

Social stress can make people sicker. People with fewer social connections are more likely to develop an illness, like cardiovascular disease. Social standing of her or him is to suffer from gastrointestinal, cardiovascular or gastrointestinal, neoplastic renal or any other chronic illness. These connections aren't accounted for by other traditional risk factors such as access, health habits such as age, gender or race when it comes to health care. Researchers conducted interviews with participants to determine whether they were experiencing conflicts or close friendships with family members. They then exposed them to the common cold virus. They Also, they found that people who had conflicting relationships were twice as likely be diagnosed with the common cold than people without societal stress. Social support, especially in regards to relief from socioeconomic migraines is ininversely linked with significant morbidity. Studies that examined the social factors that affect health in a city slum in India found that social exclusion as well as stress and a low social support are correlated to diseases, including coronary heart disease, hypertension and diabetes.

Long-Term Consequences

Youth stress can lead to increased risk of developing disease in the future and long-term effects. In particular, people who were victimized (mentally or physically, sexually neglected, or abused) as children experience more health-related outcomes, including heart attack, stroke Heart attacks, diabetic and hypertension, and even their severity. In the Adverse Childhood Experiences Study (ACE) that includes over 17 million people found that there was an increase of 20 percent in the likelihood of suffering from heart disease due to every type of family stressor that's frequently experienced by young people that wasn't due to risks that are typical for Heart conditions like hypertension or demographics.

Retrieval, and yet another ailment

Social stress has been linked with health issues. If there was a negative relationship with their spouses while adjusting the severity of illness and treatments, patients with end-stage renal disorders were at greater risk. Also, they were more likely to be affected if they were under moderate or extreme strain to suffer another incident. This result remained even after taking into account the severity of the disease, health behavior as well as demographics. With regards to HIV/AIDS, the progression could alter the course of the virus to the disease. Studies have revealed that men with HIV with more stressful life events, stress in the social and a lack of societal aid in advancing towards the clinical AIDS diagnosis more quickly than males with HIV who do not suffer from the same levels of stress from society. Females with HIV who have acquired an infection with the HSV virus, stress is a major risk factor for the spread of esophageal herpes.

Physiology

Social stress causes several modifications that regulate its relationship to health of the body. In the short-term the physiological changes described below are flexible, since they enable our nervous system cope with stress better. The inability to regulate manipulations within the long-term effects of the systems mentioned could be detrimental to health.

Sympathetic Nervous System

The sympathetic nervous system (SNS) is activated in the reaction to stress. Sympathetic stimulation triggers the medulla the medulla to release norepinephrine and epinephrine into blood vessels. This reduces the response. Perspiration increases, heart rate and blood pressure constrict so that the heart can beat and arteries dilate due to the added weight, and the flow of blood to the various parts of the body that are involved in the fight or flight reaction decreases. If this continues for the long-term and blood stress remains high, it can lead to which leads to hypertension and hypertension that are both factors that can lead to the development of disease. A variety of animal and human studies have confirmed that the risk of negative health effects rises. Research on rodents has revealed that hypertension is due to atherosclerosis and stress. Research on anti-inflammatory primates show that arteries block. While humans aren't able to be randomly assigned to be subjected to social stress due to moral issues however, research has demonstrated that bad social interactions that are characterized by combat result in increased blood pressure and heart rates. Social stress that is triggered by perceived discrimination in daily life can be associated with higher levels of blood pressure throughout the day and with a lack of blood stress dropping at night.

Hypothalamic-Pituitary Adrenocortical Axis (Hpa)

The hypothalamus releases Corticotropin-releasing hormone (CRH), stimulating the anterior pituitary gland to release adrenocorticotropic hormone (ACTH). ACTH increases the activity of adrenal glands. Social stress can result in interfering with an HPA mechanism or making it activate the HPA axis. There are numerous studies linking the signs of stress and an impaired HPA axis. For instance the monkey infants have long-lasting responses following events. For people, there is a higher level of Cortisol after a standard stressor in the laboratory is significantly higher than those who have no history of abuse. Children have higher cortisol levels in the morning levels than children. Their HPA systems aren't able to recover after interactions with their caregivers. As time passes, children show cortisol's production. The study didn't reveal any health-related outcomes, even although these studies suggest an issue with the HPA system bookkeeping that could be a reason for the relationship between stress and health. However the HPA reaction to stress may raise the chance of causing or exacerbating diseases such as cancer, hypertension, obesity, cardiovascular disease and diabetes.

Infection

Inflammation is fighting off conditions and repair of damaged tissue. While inflammation is flexible but chronic inflammation can result in negative health effects such as hypertension, diabetes and coronary heart disease hypertension, depression, and some cancers. The research has revealed a link between various Social stressors and the cytokines (the characteristic for inflammation). Social stressors that persist, such as the caregiving of spouses who has dementia, can trigger higher levels of interleukin-6, a cytokine (IL-6) as well as the intense stressors that a society experiences in laboratory studies have shown to trigger increases in proinflammatory cytokines. In addition, when faced by the other type of stress in society especially societal, participants experienced an improvement in IL-6 and an soluble receptor for tumor necrosis factor A. Inflammation are able to persist over time because studies have shown that chronic stress to connect is associated with higher production of IL-6 after six months and children raised in stress-filled family environments triggered by conflict and negligence often show elevated levels of lipoic protein, which is a indicator of IL-6 levels, into adulthood.

Interactions Of Bodily Systems

There is evidence to suggest that the physiological One another's effects have results. For instance, cortical can exert a calming influence on processes, and cytokines could also trigger HPA. HPA system. The sympathetic activity could increase the activity of inflammation. Due to the connections between these physiological mechanisms, social Stress could also affect health indirectly, by impacting one particular physiological system that in turn affects a specific physiological system.

Social Stress at Work

As organizations experience cuts to budgets, cuts to workforce reduction, it's easy to realize that workplaces can be stressful. Many of us are aware that stress can cause many concerns for our well-being and health, but we also know it's impossible to prevent all sources of Stress. Particular types that cause stress (i.e. anxiety related to deadlines or difficult tasks) are difficult to eliminate since we aren't able to simply shift deadlines or make complicated tasks easier, however other forms or stress (i.e. Social Stress) can be dealt with.

Social Stress

Social stressors are defined as situations and behavior which are connected to physical and mental stress. Examples of stressors in society include:

Affronting verbally from customers or supervisors

A fight between co-workers

Negative group surroundings

Organizational politics
Unfair treatment

Social stressors' knowledge could cause a range of results that are counter to a variety of most desirable outcomes and behaviours. The reason for this is that stressors from society deplete our ability to work (or the capacity to cope to Stress). Studies have clearly demonstrated that social stressors are the main cause of these outcomes:

Lower Job Satisfaction
More turnover
Feelings of inadequacy
Reduced productivity (because of time spent dealing with 'scenarios')
Reduced altruism and corporate citizenship behaviour (i.e. aiding employees in their office)

Reducing Social Stress

While it is true that migraines cannot be prevented The good information is that there are measures that can be undertaken to lessen the negative effects of Stress. Below is a list of the activities that could, when devoted to, help reduce stress within the community and the negative consequences that go along with it to it:

For the pioneers: stop feeling of unjust or unfair treatment by being aware of your actions. Be sure to portray yourself as a person who is fair and a and effective leader (offer feedback to everyone and be accessible) instead of picking the most popular.

For everyone: help establish guidelines for coworkers' aggression. Be aware that not all types of conflicts are eliminated (e.g. disagreements over how to do a certain task). But, social conflict is generally negative and can result in social stress. Avoid social conflict by ensuring that the discussions are based on work rather than on individual.

For HR leaders and leaders for hiring new employees be honest about the presence of social stressors in the workplace. The research shows that self-evaluations of the heart are a significant factor in how workers react to migraines. Self-evaluations of self-esteem, self-efficacy and psychological stability controller. All of these are quantifiable using assessment tools.

Chapter 11: The Way to Stop Sleeping While Thinking

It is often difficult to put your brain to sleep and get a good night's rest, as your mind is always going and around, reminiscing about what happened throughout the day. In certain instances, you start revisiting old memories, specifically those which make you feel look embarrassed.

If you're always having this racing thought within your mind it could be a sign of psychological health problems (like anxiety and stress). These types of events can occur to anyone from time to moment and do not necessarily mean you are suffering from a mental disorder Sometimes you may be experiencing a challenging period that is likely to disappear.

Every situation is unique and therefore, some methods may not be suitable for you, and you may have to look at more than one until you can find the perfect one that will help you rest more comfortably.

1. Sleep-related overthinking is a More Common occurrence

Our brains are intricate machines. They are at the central point of all bodily activity. The brain is always working.

Information is processed continuously and any slight disturbance can cause a massive impact upon your physical.

The results of studies have shown that approximately 35% of people have "poor" as well as "reasonable" quality of sleep (rated on their own) while about 25% say they aren't able to get up refreshed. These findings have led researchers to look into the possibility that insufficient sleep could lead to a major health issue.

Anxiety is one of the major factors that contribute to poor sleep or sleep deprivation and is an increasing problem in our society. This is a result of the notion of a condition of anxiety and fear about the future, the numerous or insufficient alternatives, resulting from the anticipation of actual or perceived threats, as well as situations that affect your physical and psychological health. People who are overthinking while they sleep tend to be concerned regarding their personal lives. They constantly anxious about what the future holds.

2.Health Conditions that Cause Sleep Disorders: Other than the stress factor, there's a variety of sleep-related health problems that make it difficult for people to get enough sleeping. There are illnesses that be common or uncommon.

Sleepiness is the most frequent health issue that causes sleep issues; it's caused by elevated tension, medications and anxiety, depression or alcohol or drug use. The condition can make going to sleep more difficult. It is possible to occur every now and then but when it occurs repeatedly in a row, it could become a persistent issue and need psychiatric help. The treatment is the modification of behavior or medications. A third of the population suffers from sleep issues.

Sleep apnea is caused due to a partial blockage of the throat. This causes breathing to stop for brief intervals while sleeping. The result is sleep snoring. This is the reason that most people find out that they suffer from sleep apnea because their family members tell their stories of their snoring that keeps them awake in the midnight. Along with snoring, sleep apnea is also responsible for fatigue all day long, headaches in the morning and a feeling of being constantly tired. Sleep apnea can be addressed by using an CPAP (Continuous Positive Airway Pressure) device that maintains the throat of the patient

It is open and produces a constant and consistent flow of air. There are other procedures that can be performed but don't yield similar results. Around one in five adult suffers one type of sleep apnea.

The syndrome of restless legs is a condition for which experts aren't sure of the cause Some believe it is a genetic issue while others suggest that the cause is the use of certain medications. The condition is commonly seen in women who are pregnant, which makes doctors wonder if it's caused by hormonal problems. It is defined by the need to move legs (mainly leg muscles) which is typically experienced over intervals of sleep, forcing people to kick or move their legs hundreds of times in a night. Experts suggest doing regular exercises, and also reduce alcohol and caffeine in your diet. In extreme cases, medication may be prescribed to treat other symptoms that are severe. Around 90% of population is affected by this disease and, as it is stated, is the most prevalent in women.

Rapid Eye Movement

This type of sleep disorder is a different medical condition that can cause problems in being unable to fall asleep for some individuals. REM (Rapid Eye movement) is a method that prevents movement during asleep when suffering from the disorder. It's a system that isn't working exactly as it is supposed to. Most people experience sudden and severe movements while trying to sleep. Since it's an uncommon circumstance (about 1percent of the population in the world suffers from it) The most well-known treatment is medication, however it is best to be supervised by a physician.

You may know someone who (or that previously did) sleepwalk. The condition could have a variety of reasons, but it is often caused through lack of sleep or poor quality sleep. Some drugs or illnesses can cause it to occur. Sleepwalkers walk while asleep and some do their regular activities during the day and then go back to bed. at other times, they get up during something they don't realize they did; which can result in low quality sleep, and people often feel exhausted for days following. Nobody knows the most effective method to treat this type of condition. However, doctors recommend reducing the amount of liquid consumed before bed and ensuring that you rest in a calm and peaceful space. A regular schedule for sleep is also a possibility to avoid these kinds of attacks. The condition is more common in children however, nobody has a explanation for why this happens. Certain researchers have confirmed that it's related to developing the brain, and specifically, the distinction between two different stages of sleeping (light as well as deep) and children can are prone to falling into an ambiguous state that causes them to sleepwalk.

You may be exhausted from your day-to-day life, and you're exhausted and unable to rest. It's hard to perform at a high level throughout the day if you're not getting enough rest in the evening and aren't able to recharge. This results in stress and tension and anxiety. Here are some suggestions to help you get more restful and peaceful nights of sleep.

3. Techniques to Stop Thinking While sleeping

Sleeping while thinking is a major battle. It can be difficult to address difficulties in falling asleep since people aren't aware of the cause and the best way to treat the issues naturally.

Take a break from the daily Stress and calm Your Mind

One of the major issues faced by those who are unable to not stop thinking during sleep is that they have an active mind.

Being creative and active is usually a great asset at work, and also for your life and career all around. However in the evening, when trying to sleep the constantly active mind can become very disruptive.

It wouldn't be a problem when people can easily fall asleep following an extended day at work. Our minds need the right mix of both activity and sleep - and sleep comes in the evening as we fall asleep. If you find it difficult to relax and drift asleep, it will assist you to keep free of bright light sources and stay clear of any type of screen (tablets or phones, computer system, television) since these devices could fool your brain into thinking that it's still daylight and that it's not the right time to take a nap. Find methods to calm the body and mind and assist in allowing your brain to begin closing down naturally.

We offer methods to calm your mind to assist you in falling asleep and have an improved night's sleep.

1. Establish a pre-sleeping regimen

Many people who have this disorder struggle to shut their minds as it relates to the time of going to bed. Because of our busy lifestyle our brains are engaged throughout the day, right up to time to go to bed. The issue is that our minds must be able to rest in order to enable easy to sleep. In order to begin this process, you must be following a sleep routine prior to bedtime that assists your body to recognize that it's time to unwind from the stress-inducing activities. To achieve more effective results, your routine should begin around thirty minutes (or more) prior to bedtime and should include at least one (or several) activities that allow you to relax such as doing yoga, reading and listening to calming music, or watching a relaxing show. We suggest that you stay clear of the use of screens during this method, since they can put your brain in the "active" state, which makes it difficult to relax.

2.Is your head overflowing with thoughts, ideas, information, questions or worries, agendas for the coming days, etc? Note them all down! Take them out of your mind to paper and that you can fall asleep with a clear, calm mind. Recording what's going through your mind before going to bed can help relax your mind and is a great method for eliminating anxiety. Once you rid of your mind of the tangle of thoughts that engulfed it, it'll be simpler to drift off to sleep. 3. Breathe through your left nostril

It may sound a bit odd, but breathing through your left nostril could aid in relaxing your nervous system, easing your imagination and mind greatly increasing your ability to sleep naturally and completely to sleep. For this method it is necessary to close your right nostril by using the thumb of your right hand and then take a longbreathing deep breath through your left nostril. Hold and exhale, repeating the process in order to eliminate anxiety and stress.

stress from your body and help let your mind relax simultaneously.

4. Spend some time reading

Reading can be a beneficial activity that helps to relax your body up, as well as calm your mind at the same at the same time. Of course, it will depend on the content you're reading. So take note of the right books or articles that won't stimulate your mind. Read something that is tranquil, relaxing or soothing and leave anything exciting frightening, political or similar for your afternoon reading.

5. Meditate

Meditation can help relax your mind and your body. However, only when it's done properly. It is suggested to concentrate on each breath and do it slowly. By doing this, you'll lower your heart rate, calming your body and mind. Relax and enjoy your meditation practice. rid your mind of issues and thoughts, and then unwind your muscles. When you've meditated you'll be able to fall asleep faster and will rest more completely.

6. Enjoy relaxing music

Relaxing music is a great way to relax. It will allow your mind to be calm and relaxed. By focusing on these relaxing songs, your mind is diverted from other ideas.

7. Don't be so eager to be relaxed!

If you're trying different ways to relax and calm your mind so that it can fall asleep but you're trying to settle your mind, when these strategies aren't effective, then relax and stop trying too for so long! Sometimes, trying to achieve results can have an opposite result and results in frustration for you, and increases your chances of falling asleep. If you notice that one strategy doesn't perform for you, try another ... Always look for other methods until you have found the most efficient approach for you. Also, you should seek out the assistance from an expert should there is no solution, or if you suffer from an illness that affects your health.

Focus On Mental Imagery

From an early age you may have been instructed to count sheep if you're having trouble sleeping, and you could

You may think that this is completely ineffective and absurd, but, in reality is when you are focused on something other than what is distracting you, it may assist you in ignoring the issues for a sufficient amount of time that you can relax and receive adequate sleep. Certain experts recommend repeating simple words such as "the" inside your brain. The continuous repetition of letters and the sound can reduce the amount of energy your brain produces and reduce the stress which is making it difficult in relaxing. If you can put aside your thoughts, you are able to properly rest...Here are some strategies that you can employ to bring your imaginative imagination to life, helping ease your mind.

1. Envision

If you are experiencing an overly creative mind, you need to gain from it in order to stop the excessive thinking while you sleep. Imagine an enchanted scene as if you are a leaf carried by a gentle breeze or you're being sucked into a smooth cloud. Visualize scenes that loosen up will help you get your mind distracted from problems and emotional thoughts.

2. It is a way of counting things.

It is possible that you have observed, thinking that when you were a kid, and counting sheep could be an easy method to sleep better as engaging the mind with regular mental exercises will help relax your mind, and as being calming for your mind.

3. Alphabetize

One simple way to make use of your imagination and unwind your body is to do a mental workout which distracts your brain and promotes sleep. For instance to Go through the alphabet, and then count out products for each letter.

4. Take a picture of something

Focus on something specific: Imagine the shade, dimensions, shape, how each dimension appears and how it is used. It is also possible to imagine a scene. imagine you're biking or walking, imagine the street, the area houses, roads and so on.

As best you do. The more information you can think of, the greater it will be for you.

5. Recite rhymes, quotes, or lyrics

A great psychological activity to keep your mind occupied is to sing the lyrics of your favourite track or quoting from your most loved movie. This technique helps your mind concentrate on something specific , which will help relax your mind and aid in sleeping.

6. Create stories with your mind

Writing stories is a great method of keeping your mind active and imagining the people as well as the things and places in your head and ask yourself: What's you character up to? What is his/her location? What would the scene look like? If you are having trouble thinking of a character could imagine yourself in a different situation which relaxes you.

Release Your Body

If your body is at ease and relaxed, it's easier to fall asleep The anxiety and stress disappears and you are relaxed.

enough to allow you to drift off in bed. Certain situations that you're concerned about could create stress for your body, that you'll have trouble getting to bed. Therefore it is possible that unwinding your body can be the solution to your problem:

1. The temperature level is reduced of your body

One of the primary reasons that you are unable to relax is because the temperature of your body is high. Therefore, one method to help you rest is to reduce the body temperature. You can either reduce the temperature of your room and/or eliminate blankets to keep you cool. The ideal room temperature is between 15 to 25 Celsius (about 60-75 Fahrenheit).

2. Take a warm and relaxing bath

If your room is not at the recommended temperature it is possible that you require a bath to raise your body's temperature so that, when you get into your bed, the temperature of your body decreases and eventually reduces the metabolic rate that causes you to be exhausted. It is also possible to apply aromatherapy while bathing to create

the use of products that have scents such as lavender and chamomile , which have properties that soothe.

3. Workout

Exercise is great for you. It improves your overall health and wellbeing it strengthens your muscles, helps prevent diseases and improves your body and mind, resulting in a better sleep. Do your best to workout for around three hours before you go to bed.

4. Take a deep breath

Make sure to take more time to breathe out rather than breathe in. Also, stop between breaths. Taking deep breaths can relax you deeply. I recommend sitting on the floor before you go to bed , turning off the lights and focusing on your breathing by using this technique you'll clear your mind and relax your body.

5. Take hot tea

Certain plants possess relaxing properties that make them a great choice for those who have trouble when they want to relax. The use of lavender, valerian or chamomile tea could help you.

aids in sleeping more easily. There is no need to add sugar in your drink in order to sleep better, considering that it may cause you to stay awake.

6.Get more sunlight during the entire day. The sun's rays causes the brain to alter its internal clock, making it easier to fall asleep at night. Professional athletes utilize this technique to guarantee their efficiency when they travel or compete in other countries They attempt to receive as much sunlight exposure as they can in the morning to avoid jet-lag. Although you may not be an elite athlete, but in order to enjoy a an enjoyable night's rest it is possible to use the techniques and strategies of professional athletes. Make sure you take advantage of as much light exposure as possible in the morning to give your body the chance to get a later sleep.

Get rid of any noise in your Bedroom

The setting where you sleep is one of the major elements that determine your capacity to sleep or not. It is essential to take extreme attention to certain aspects of your sleeping environment, which can directly impact your capacity to rest. Small changes to your everyday activities can make huge differences:

1. Limit the amount of light entering your bedroom.

The light from the outside keeps the body awake, which disrupts the regular cycle of your circadian (the biological process that displays an internal, continuous 24 hour oscillation). You must stop using all electronic devices about an hour before you go to bed, so that your body will begin producing Melatonin.

2. Reduce your consumption of caffeine

Many people drink coffee to remain awake for a long period of time so that they are able to accomplish their goals. We recommend that you limit your the consumption of coffee since it is high in caffeine (a powerful stimulant). However, certain kinds of tea (such such as teas that are black) are also rich in caffeine and should be avoided at all times. be careful not to drink them before bedtime.

3. You should only go to bed in the event that you're worn out:

Another reason why people are awake in the night is because they are unable to get to bed, even though their bodies are not rested enough.

It is possible to even. If you are going to bed at night, and do not need to sleep can result in continuous turning and twirling all night long as your mind continues to be twisted and turned by thoughts. If it takes you longer than 20 minutes before falling asleep, you must take a break and attempt to unwind before you go to sleep.

4. Making use of and remembering the bed as a sleeping place Instead of tossing and turning you should stand up so that your body does not remember the bed as an opportunity to get up in the event that you are unable to sleep.

Chapter 12: Mindfulness Meditation

No matter if you're contemplating the demands of work, family at school, what you're planning to cook for dinner or what you talked about at the end of last at the end of your night or any of the preceding things, it's not difficult to be caught in a twirling set of thoughts. Every now and then, we think about the past, sometimes in a way that causes anxiety, or we think about the possible outcomes of events to be.

Mindfulness-based reflection is a psychotherapeutic training practice that can be helpful in these conditions. It helps you bring your thoughts into the present moment, while focusing on the thoughts, feelings and feelings you're experiencing "in the present moment." Although it may initially be difficult to settle your thoughts With time and effort, you'll be able to experience the benefits of mindful reflection, which include less stress and anxiety and even a decrease in the symptoms of conditions such as IBS.

Mindfulness-related systems may change but as a general rule mindfulness reflection involves meditation practice meditation, mental symbolism and a sense of familiarity with the body and mind as well as body and muscle unwinding.

The first step to begin a meditation practice is to start with Mindfulness.

One of the first formalized initiatives for mindfulness meditation can be found in the Mindfulness Based Stress Reduction (MBSR) program, which is an study under the supervision that is a study of Buddhist religious priests and researchers Thich Nhat Hanh. The program, which runs for eight weeks, guides students to be present moment, decrease emotions and reactivity, and attain a state that is peaceful. The other, more confused, common mindfulness meditations are being progressively integrated into therapeutic environments to treat depression, stress, and pain among various ailments.

It is easy enough to practice on your own but instructors or programs can assist you in beginning with the practice, particularly if you're practicing meditation for explicit health motives. Although some people think for long periods of time, even few minutes of constant reflection can result in any impact. Here's a crucial approach to guide you in getting started:

1. Find a calm and comfortable location. You can sit in a chair or on the ground with your neck, head and back straight, but not firmly. It's also helpful to wear a loose-fitting shirt to ensure you're not engaged.

2. Try to forget any thoughts of the future and memories and concentrate upon the current.

3. Become conscious of your breathing, and adjust to the sound of the air that is moving through your body while you lay back. Notice your stomach rising and fall as you let air move through your noses before it go out of your mouth. Pay attention to the way your breath changes with each breath and is distinctive.

4.Watch every thought go forward and back regardless of whether it's an anxiety, stress or tension. When thoughts arise in your mind Don't ignore or suppress them. Simply note them down, remain still, and use your breathing to grapple.

5.If you find yourself becoming excessively focused on your concerns take note of where your thoughts are was going, with no judgement, and come back to your calming. Remember that you shouldn't be a burden to yourself in the event of this happening.

6.As the chance arises near you, take a moment or two, and try to be aware of the place you are. Take a step back slowly.

Incorporating Mindfulness into Your Everyday Life

There's no law that states that you must take a seat in a calm area to practice the art of mindfulness, claims Kate Hanley, creator of "A Year of Daily Calm." Meditation is one method but regular workouts and projects provide plenty of opportunities to practice.

Here are Hanley's suggestions for improving your mindfulness throughout your day everyday routine.

Cleaning the Dishes

Have you ever noticed that no one is trying to make themselves stand out enough to be noticed when you're making the dishes? The combination of time alone and monotonous physical movements makes cleaning up after dinner to be an exceptional opportunity to practice some mindfulness. Relax and enjoy the feeling of warm water that is soaking your fingers, the sound from the pockets of air, and the reflection of the dish that is thumping on the floor of your sink.

Zen instructor Thich Nhat Hanh describes this practice "washing dishes to wash them"and not to finish them off and done so that you can to the television. When you are able to surrender completely to this experience you'll get the mental refreshment as well as an uncluttered kitchen.

Cleaning Your Teeth

There's no way to go for a single day without cleaning your teeth, which makes this an ideal opportunity to practice your mindfulness. Begin by imagining your feet planted on the ground with the brush in your hand and your arms moving across.

Driving

It's not difficult to ponder your thoughts while driving and thinking about what you'd like to make for dinner or what you forgot to accomplish at work the previous day. Make use of your focus to ensure that your thoughts are restricted to the confines of your vehicle. The radio can be a mood killer, or put on something that is relaxing like the old-fashioned music. As you imagine your spine getting taller Find the midpoint between loosening your hands and gripping the steering wheel too tightly at any point you notice your mind wandering you should return your focus to the point where you and your car are located in the world.

Training

The thought of sitting watching the TV while you run on the treadmill could make your workout go faster but it doesn't bring much peace to your mind. Relax both your mental and physical muscles by removing all screens and focusing on your breathing and the position of your feet are while you move.

Making preparations for bed Bedtime

Instead of rushing through your evening schedule and fighting with your children during the time to sleep, try to take the time to truly enjoy the experience. Reach a similar to your children's level gaze into their eyes, pay attention longer than you speak and take pleasure in any cuddles. As soon as you stop the curtains, they will also.

Mindfulness is the human ability to be fully present, aware of the place we're in and what we're up to, and not overly attentive or overwhelmed by what's happening in the world around us.

It's not just in your head. You can learn mindfulness by sitting down for a traditional meditation practice, or by becoming more deliberate and aware of the activities you do each day.

If you're looking to learn more about mindfulness and the best way to practice mindfulness meditation, check out the Getting Started page.

The most efficient way to practice Mindfulness when you are in a rush

Each task we undertake during the day, whether it's cleaning our teeth or eating lunch, talking to friends or going to the gym--should be achievable with greater care.

As we're conscious of our actions and are aware of our actions, we pay more attention to what we're doing. It's not like doing nothing at all. Instead it is a focus on your thoughts, observing your thoughts and emotions.

When you incorporate mindfulness into your day to every day routine, you can practice mindfulness in any situation even when you're too busy to think about meditation.

Finding out the best way to meditate

The first time you do it you will be able to set a time of time you will not doubt its "practice" to. Or, you can focus on the time when you should end. If you're just beginning with an initial time frame such as five or 10 minutes. It is inevitable that you will grow to double the length and, in the end, up to 30 minutes, 45 or even 60 minutes. Use a kitchen clock or the one that you have on your mobile. A lot of people have a timer in the early part of the day, and later at the night, or both. When you feel like that your life is busy and you are only able to stay for a short time that shows improvement over the same thing. When you are able to see a bit of reality, you'll be able to achieve more.

Find a suitable spot in your home in a perfect world , where there's not a lot of chaos and where you can find peace. Turn off the lights or just sit in the light of the common. You may also sit outside whenever you'd like but choose a place without interruption.

The stance is a great start of a time of contemplation or to do something for a short time, perhaps to get your balance and see a glimpse of unwinding before returning to the battle. If you're dealing with injuries or physical issues it is possible to modify the exercises to fit your needs.

Step-by-step directions to sit for Mindfulness Meditation

1.Take Your seat. Whatever you're sitting on, a seat or a reflection pad an exercise center seat--find the sign that will give you a stable, solid seat. You're not roosting or waiting.

2.Notice the movements you're doing with your legs. When you are on a mat placed on the floor make sure you fold your legs in a way before you. (And once you are doing some kind of standing yoga pose, move on.) If you're sitting on a chair it's great if soles of your feet are touching the floor.

3.Straighten--yet don't slam your chest. The spine has a regular flow and ebb. Give it a chance be there. Your shoulders and head can rest comfortably on your vertebrae.

4.Situate your arms in a parallel position to your chest. When you are there, you can let your hands fall to the top that your legs are. While your arms are in your side your hands will land at the right position. If you are too far forward, it can cause you to look like you're hunched over. A lot of backwards will cause you to become firm. Your body is tuning the strings of your body, which isn't very tight and not very supple.

5.Drop your jawline and let your eyes drop slowly downwards. You can let your lower your eyes. If you are feeling that you need to, you can lower them completely but it's not necessary to shut your eyes while looking back. It is possible to let whatever is visible to your eyes without being focused on it.

6.Be in the area for couple of minutes. Unwind. Concentrate on your breath or the sensations that are in your body.

7.Feel your breath or some other states "pursue" it--as it flows out and into. (A several variations of this method place more emphasis on the outbreath and for the inbreath, just let a little delay.) Whatever you choose, force yourself to be aware of the physical effects of breathing, the air flowing through your mouth or nose or mouth, the rising and fall of your midsection as well as your chest. Find your point of convergence and as you breathe you will be able to rationally observe "taking into" in and "breathing out."

8.Inevitably your mind will depart from your breath and drift off to other locations. Be careful not to overthink it. There's no reason that you should cut off or stop thinking. When you begin to see your mind wandering in a short time, perhaps a second five minutes or less--just gently take a second to reflect on your breath.

9.Practice waiting a while the moment you make any physical changes, such as movement of your body or even rubbing your tense. While aiming, move for the pace you prefer and allow space between your experience and the actions you choose to take.

10.You might find your mind wandering around in a constant loop, which is normal and also. Instead of trying to figure out or absorbing the thoughts to that extent, try to see without expecting to be able to respond. Just sit and concentrate. If you find it difficult in order to maintain your pace, that's all that is important. Repeat the process without judging or desire.

11. When you're ready, gently move your gaze (if your eyes are closed or closed, let them open). Pay attention to any sounds you hear on the earth. Pay attention to how your body feels now. Be aware of your thoughts and feelings. After a brief stop, decide what you'd like to do in your day.

This is the end of it. That's the instruction. It's been said often that it's easy, but it's actually not easy. The trick is to continue to do it. The results will be gathered.

OTHER MEDITATION TECHNIQUES

There are alternative methods of contemplation. One example is a typical day daily practice of contemplation among Buddhist priests is centered around the cultivation of empathy. This involves imagining events that are negative and then recasting them in positive light through changing the situation through compassion. There are also moving contemplation methods, such as yoga, qigong and walking contemplation .

The benefits of a good EDITATION

Unwinding isn't an goal of contemplation, it is often a result. In the 1970s, Herbert Benson, MD, an analyst at Harvard University Medical School, invented the phrase "unwinding reaction" after leading research on people who practiced the art of the process of contemplation that is thought to be supernatural. The unwinding response, in Benson's terms"is "an inverted, automatic reaction that causes a reduction in the actions of the brain's sensor."

The goal of reflection is to focus and to comprehend your mind, ultimately arriving at a higher degree of inner calm and mindfulness. Reflection is a quaint method, but researchers are still discovering all of its benefits. Regular reflection can help you in regulating your emotions and improve your focus decrease stress and develop a deeper connection with the those in your vicinity. Through learning, you'll have an possibility of achieving a sense of peace and harmony regardless of the events around you. There are many ways to consider, and when one approach doesn't seem to be effective for you, try another method that is better for you prior to deciding to give up.

Different types of meditation

Meditation is a general term used to describe the various methods to attain a relaxed state of being. There are a variety of unwinding and contemplation methods which include reflection elements. Each has the goal of achieving inner harmony.

Methods of ruminating can include:

Guided contemplation. It is sometimes referred to as symbolic representation or guided symbolism, by using this method for reflection you create mental images of the places or events that you observe unraveling.

Try to utilize as you can as appropriate, including the smells, sights, and even surfaces. You may be guided through this process by a teacher or guide.

Mantra reflection. In this type of reflection you recite an unspoken word, thought , or expression to keep your thoughts from diverting.

Mindfulness meditation. This kind of contemplation is based on mindfulness or having a greater awareness of the present moment and being aware of what is happening today.

When you meditate you increase your awareness and awareness. Concentrate on what you notice during your contemplation, like the movement of your breath. It is possible to watch your thoughts and emotions, but allow them to go without judgement.

Qi gong. The training in general involves unwinding, reflection breathing and physical training to help restore and preserve the harmony. The Qi Gong (CHEE-gung) is one component of traditional Chinese drug.

Judo. It is a form of delicate Chinese hand-to-hand combat. Judo (TIE-CHEE) you will carry with a self-guided sequence of stances or movements in a gentle, graceful method while practicing deep relaxation.

Supernatural Meditation(r). Supernatural Meditation is a simple routine method. In Transcendental Meditation, you consciously repeat a by and by repeated mantra, such as the word, sound or phrase, keeping an end goal in mind.

This type of meditation can allow your body to relax to a state of profound relaxation and unwinding, and also your mind to attain an internal peace and harmony, without the need to use focus or effort.

Yoga. You practice a variety of stances , controlled breathing to build an ever-changing body and a peaceful personality. While you move through scenes that require fixation and equalization You're encouraged to focus less on the whirlwind of your schedule and instead focus on your moment.

Chapter 13: Stress Management for Parents

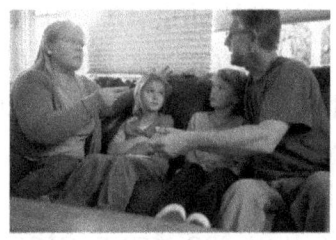

Parental stress , also known as "parenting stress" refers to a numb feeling that you feel towards yourself as well as your child. The sensation is experienced abruptly that you attribute it to pressures that are imposed by the role of parents. Most parents suffer from this kind of anxiety. It's true that parenting can be extremely stressful. While you may want to remain calm and at peace constantly, if your children are acting out in a situation stressing, it's difficult to achieve that. Since you aren't able to completely eliminate stress and anxiety completely from your life The next step is to figure out how to lessen or manage it.

Today, stress for parents can be caused by many different things. Anything from an infant who is refusing to eat dinner, to something as large as the child who throws a tantrum in public could cause parents stress. And the amount of stress you experience would differ from the stress levels you feel from other parents you are familiar with. The first thing to remember is to not look at yourself in comparison to other parents. It will cause stress. Instead, concentrate on your own and how you can handle every stressful experience with the greatest efficiency.

Characteristics of Parental Stress

As parents, you are required to face questions that you must solve, issues you have to solve, or even a kiss you have to kiss, choices you have to take, and many other similar issues every day. These things could result in some degree of stress, based on how well you're capable of handling these issues. If you don't want to wind in a state of being broken or burned out, you need to be able to identify the symptoms of parental stress.

Alongside dealing with your own issues, being anxious at work, conflict that you have with your husband, problems with your family members, and other things, you need to take care of the children, nurture them and ensure that your child grows into a balanced adult. When you face stress, you're also teaching your child to handle anxiety with grace and competence. This is why it's so crucial to know how to manage stress in the home in a more effective manner. In the event that you don't, your child could become a victim of what they consider to be "wrong ways," and you don't want to see that occur. Let's examine the most common signs of stress in the home so that you're aware of them once you begin to notice these within yourself. You feel exhausted constantly

If you're experiencing parents' stress it can feel like you're never able to get your energy back. If someone asks you what you think as a parent, your first answer will be "tired." No matter how much sleep you get in the time of night or how many napping sessions you take throughout each day, this fatigue you feel won't disappear. The reason is that stress from parents takes away your energy. If you don't learn to handle it, that's the way you'll feel every day.

It can be a nightmare to sleep for those who sleep.

It's one reason you're tired all the time, and it's because you're not sleeping enough. Because of the stress that parents face Your mind is always racing. Your mind is constantly thinking about all the things you need to accomplish for your kids and how you can ensure the best possible future they can have, and so on. If you're unable to get your thoughts off, this can make you feel more stressed. Whatever you'd like to sleep the stress of parenting will never cease to keep you from getting that sleep you require to survive and flourish.

This can cause you to be irritable.

If your spouse, children or any other person mentions their name to you, you respond by snippy. Stress as a parent can make you feel constantly in a state of anxiety. So, you're likely be irritable at the most insignificant things. Be cautious, since you may be screaming at your kids without even realizing it. If you find yourself overly harsh or hot-headed and irritable, you need to begin getting better at managing your stress better.

It can cause you to forget.

This can be especially apparent in mothers because there's a phenomenon known called"a "pregnant brain" or an "mommy brain" in which you've the tendency to forget things every once in some time. However, when you're overwhelmed by the demands of the mommy life, you'll be frequently being distracted by things. This is evident especially when you have sharp memories of the past. Then, suddenly, you're at a point wherein you cannot remember anything that happened prior to the current moment. It's also difficult to remember where you put crucial items when you require them most. This is another typical symptom of stress in the home which can be extremely annoying. If you're a father with this issue stress, the anger can become more acute.

It causes you to struggle when you work
It's obvious that this is the case for those who aren't giving up their career. Even if you've been successful in your career previously, stress from parenting can make you feel as if you're strugglingand find it difficult to pick yourself up. Because you're contemplating all the duties and concerns you face as a parent, you'll not be able focus on your job. In the end you may contemplate quitting in order to ease the burden. However, this isn't the best option. You're experiencing stress from your parents. Learn to manage it first. And you may discover the enthusiasm and dedication you had previously when you worked that made you excel at it.

It causes you to forget your responsibilities as a parent

The longer you let the stress of parenting to continue and you'll become apathetic to your responsibilities. If you were in the past, it is possible that might have enjoyed serving your family. You would cook five-course meals as well as read them bedtime tales and play with them and so on. Now, you're making excuses for doing other things in order to not have the burden of having to "be the parent" since it's making you feel overwhelmed. Instead, you let you to become distracted by trivial things, and leave your children to take care of themselves. And when you finally go to sleep, you are feeling ashamed because you haven't taken good care of them like you used to previously. This leads to a cycle of negative thoughts that must stop as soon as you can.

Stress for parents is a fact of daily life. It's debilitating, distracting and the longer you don't address it the more difficult it gets. The first step to do to get rid of this kind of anxiety is acknowledge that you're experiencing it. Track how stressed you are throughout your day and work to identify the circumstances which really annoy you. The more conscious you are in regards to your level of stress the better you'll be in a position to manage them. So, it's less likely to get to the point that you begin to associate the negative emotions with the parenting. To overcome the stress of parenting takes a lot of conscious effort, control of emotions, and a lot of reflection. However, all of your efforts will result in a positive outcome over time when you begin to view the role of parenting as a positive aspect to your everyday life.

Coping with Parental Stress

If you're experiencing parental stress, you require patience, support, and time and feel that people around you are aware of what you're going through and are willing to assist you. As parent, you have to feel respected and appreciated to ease the anxiety you experience. Although stress from parenting can be extremely painful, challenging and frustrating, it does not mean that you are unable to be able to overcome it. The most important thing is to understand how to manage difficult situations and to learn how be aware before you take action.

It's not a wise decision to let stress from your parents to dominate your life. This is due to the fact that this kind of stress tends to strain the entire family. The stress can cause you to lose your patience quickly and your relationships begin to break to pieces, and then you be feeling a bit depressed about one another. Are you willing to allow the same thing to occur for your loved ones? I'm sure you don't. Here are some tips to assist you in dealing with the stress of parenting.

Create healthy habits and establish Goals
The first thing to take care of for the improvement of your lifestyle is to establish healthy habits and establish positive objectives. As as a parent, you need to be the most effective role example of your child. The best way to accomplish this is to demonstrate that you're committed to your goals. The

practices you adopt will benefit your daily life. If your children are exposed to these traits while growing up, there's an increased chance that they will follow in your footsteps. This is a good thing because good habits can make you resilient enough to face anxiety, and setting goals helps you stay driven and motivated to continue moving forward regardless of the stress of parenting.

Reconsider your position and think about how you are living your current situation. When you're reading this article, there's a good chance you're dealing with stress from your parents and are looking to understand how you can handle it more effectively. If you take a look at your own daily life, you could uncover a few things you'd like to alter in order to make improvements. When you do this, you'll be able to enhance your skills in coping as well.

One thing you can begin altering to increase your health is the environment you live in. Making adjustments to your workplace (if you're a mom working) or your home, as well as your social environment could have a positive effect on your behaviour. The changes you make can also affect your stress levels and your abilities to cope with stress. In particular, if you live in a messy space it can create greater stress. If your home is cluttered and you're unable to locate anything that you require, and you are constantly bumping into things all over your house, what can you do to relax? Even if you have time off but you're not able to completely relax when you live in a mess. Make an effort to clean things up and see what the difference it makes to your life. To make it more enjoyable invite your entire family members to help clean up. This can ease anxiety and allows you to spend the time you deserve with your loved ones. Once everything is finished you'll be all happy with the work you've achieved.

Another beneficial change you could implement in your lifestyle today is to improve your diet. This is important for your family, yourself and everyone else in your family. Whatever your schedule are, ensure that you eat a healthy and balanced diet. Make sure your children are eating the same healthy lifestyle like you do. If you eat this way you're giving your body the right nutrition needed to provide you with enough energy to cope with stress effectively. Make sure you are eating whole food items that are rich in nutrients to keep you satisfied and healthy. You'll also be stronger and healthier.

If you are looking to change your lifestyle it's not necessary to be a complete jerk. It's not something that is easy. Create an outline of healthy behaviors and tackle them by one (or 2) at one time. The process of breaking the goals down (yes planning to change your behavior could make it one of the goals) can make them more feasible and feasible. Every time you're capable of changing the way you conduct yourself and feel inspired to continue.

In addition to creating goals to build healthy habits, you must also establish goals for learning how to handle stress better. You'll be learning more of these strategies as you read through this book, and you are able to incorporate them into your goals. The trick is to set goals and then maintain a greater commitment to follow through with them. Setting goals is an essential aspect of life because it builds you up and more resilient. It also makes you more prepared to handle stress.

Get More Sleep

A good night's sleep is crucial as it helps to ease the strain you experience all day. Did you have a time when you stayed up late for a few days in the same time? If yes, then you could be feeling tired, uneasy or even anxious. Imagine if you were to encounter your triggers for stress when you feel the same way. Naturally, the stress you feel due to these triggers is significantly greater than the stress you'd experience in a state of relaxation, rest and focused. If you're experiencing poor sleep routines, it can make life much more difficult. If you're experiencing sleep issues or aren't able to get enough rest every night, it's time to alter your sleeping habits.

When stress from parents is a major stressor and you feel that you're lacking the strength to cope and you feel anxious, angry and so on. The more you experience these feelings more, the more they activate the stress circuits in your brain. If this happens it can be hard to sleep and remain in bed all night. In essence, this means that if you're stressed, it's difficult to fall asleep. If you're unable to sleep properly, you're unable to manage stress. This leads to a vicious, hazardous cycle that could cause you to burn out as a mother.

This shouldn't occur. Therefore, it is important to ensure that you are sleeping at a regular time. Similar to how you create a routine for bedtime for your kids, you should create an evening routine for yourself and also. While you get them ready to go to bed, you can do the restorative things alongside them. For example, when your children brush their teeth, you should brush your own teeth as well. If you are reading your children a story before bed Take this opportunity to unwind to let your thoughts drift down. By doing this, it makes it simpler to get ready to go to bed. After following this routine for a certain amount of duration, your body will get familiar with it. When you finish the bedtime routine of your kids, you'll begin to feel sleepy also.

Children need to sleep in order to develop and grow normally, you too require enough sleep to function effectively. It is important to not ignore this aspect of your daily life if you are looking to improve your ability to handle stress of parenting.

Don't Overthink It!

Being too focused is among the negative behaviors you need to break. Concentrating on and worrying about worrying about things that are stressful can take you to the brink of despair, and even lead to you aging at an earlier rate! Try to not think too much. You'll find that you'll be able to accomplish more.

Imagine the following picture: A child gets sick, and it's late at night to take their child in to see a doctor. If your normal reaction to difficult situations is fret or think too much, you could create terrifying or frightening scenarios within your head. Instead of this you should simply take your child to an emergency room and have them evaluated. This is a more sensible decision that will allow you to determine what is wrong in your child. Once the doctor has diagnosed your child's condition and you know what you need to do to make your child feel better. Problem solved!

We often make ourselves stressed through overthinking rather than acting. The mind is a powerful thing. If you make use of the mind to your advantage in a destructive manner and you are stressed, the more will feel. To counter this, you might also make an effort to limit the amount of exposure you have to media that is negative. This can reduce the possibility of thinking negative thoughts. If, for instance, you spend your spare time reading reports on conflict, famine, or loss, you'll start being depressed about the world and you could develop an unhappiness mindset. If you're faced with a stressful situation, this attitude causes you to start contemplating the possibility of dire circumstances prior to trying to search for solutions. Therefore, instead of being exposed to the negatives of life find the positive side of things.

If you want to keep working well, then good for you! However, one thing you must do is not bring work home. It is commonplace to spend the majority of your time at work and if you decide to bring your stress at work home, it will impact your lifestyle. While working you're confronting your own pressures. deadlines, challenging coworkers, things you've not completed and much more. All of this does not give you the opportunity to be a good parent for your kids. When you're distracted by other things, it's impossible to remain completely with your children.

Develop a Schedule

After you've cleared your mind of worrying and overthinking, it is now time to begin planning your activities better. If you are faced with challenges and stressful circumstances, allow yourself the time to work through them. Based on the circumstances and the situation, don't try to resolve problems in a single day. This can cause you to become more stressed. Relax, your body and mind will be grateful to your for taking it.

To increase your ability to manage stress create your own routine. From the time you get up until the time you go to bed, sticking to the same routine each day will help you feel an inner peace.

Chapter 14: The Daily Affirmations

Your day should be filled with optimism, and the root of that positive energy must begin with your own self. What was the last thing that you did to yourself? Did you give yourself praise for the job you did or did you internal criticize you for failing to do it right? Do you think you would talk to your loved ones exactly the same way if you did something wrong? Perhaps not, and if not, why would you talk to yourself in that manner.

It's easy to judge yourself for a mistake you made up, or simply about the way you perceive yourself generally. A single negative thought could accumulate in your head and be a torrent of negative thoughts and nit-picking everything about you. The thought may begin with, "I do not like the way my body looks wearing this dress.' In essence, it's actually the shirt that is the issue rather than your body but what it ultimately comes down to is, 'I don't look great in anything, I'm a shite with my body. How can anyone love me?

While it may appear odd but the natural way of thinking is to be focused on tiny things until they grow into large things. It is essential to keep this in mind prior to your thoughts become too much. The mind is an fascinating thing. The brain's nervous and thought system generates habits. It develops neural pathways which become familiar to speed up the process of thinking. In the event that your thought patterns are constantly negative, the nerve pathway becomes an avenue which all your thoughts would like to travel on.

It is your responsibility to help your thoughts travel paths that go back, transforming your thoughts to positive ones, and then establishing the pathways. It starts by acknowledging your thoughts as they occur, and then making them positive. Imagine the situation as follows. If you were to communicate your thoughts on the way your body appears to your closest friend What would they say? If you told them that you're a total failure due to a blundering task at work, the person will not reply, 'Well you ought to give up because you did a horrible job'. They'd respond, "Okay there's a chance that you misjudged the project, but do you remember how successful you were with your previous project, and before that? Let's figure out a way to improve it.' You are your very own most trusted friend. You're there for your self every day. Treat yourself with the same love that your friend could give to.

You can improve your thinking by becoming more attentive to your thoughts. Your subconscious thoughts are constantly happening which is why it's your responsibility to be more conscious of the thoughts that are swirling through your mind. Start by trying to spend a few minutes every hour to reflect on your inner thoughts. Did the majority of your thoughts be negative or positive? Are your thoughts rational? The brain often allows thoughts to go way out of proportion and they are usually absurd. Keep your mind in line by let your brain's rational side decide if those thoughts are worthy of your attention.

Your thought could be "My boss is planning to dismiss me for failing the task. I'll be unable afford my loan and I'll get kicked out. I'll be forced to live with my mother and my kids will need to move schools and will hate me.' Let your rational mind come in and return you to the beginning of zero. You're not fired, and therefore you have money to pay your bills. All of your fears have come true at the moment So, calm down. Return to the initial problem, the unfinished assignment. Find a solution to resolve your issue head-on. Discuss the issue with your boss. Find a way to improve the project in order to turn into a successful one. Refraining from the issue and being fired is not a great option.

Give yourself a compliment whenever you accomplish something small. Do yourself a favor and pat yourself on the back after you've finished your dishes, put away and folded away the laundry, made it through a tough meeting, and returned to home in time. Keep in mind that even the smallest routine things are worthy of celebrating since for some people simply getting out of the bed is an accomplishment. Be aware that you're doing great, and whatever you do throughout the day should be rewarded with an applaud.

Start saying affirmations daily to yourself each day before you begin your day. The words you say within the first hour after waking to get up will set the mood for your entire day, so ensure that it's positive. When you wake up, get in bed, switch on the lights and take a look at the surroundings. It's a good thing you woke up in a good position on top of the earth So you must be grateful. Be grateful for a roof over your head and a place to lie in. You're way ahead of the curve. When you start your morning routine, pay pleasure in all your possessions. Take note of the breakfast you're eating as a gift and also as a reflection of your previous accomplishments. Be aware that your dishes, the laundry, and dishes are evidence that you have clothes and a home to live in, and food to consume.

When you are getting dressed and prepared, remember that your body has taken you to where you are today and that it's an honor. It shouldn't be judged because it is too large or having flaws. Take a look as you look in your mirror. Set the mood of the entire day. Out loud, say the affirmations you make every day:

I am strong I am here and I'm a success. I have done numerous things throughout my life and this day will be not be any different. Today I am going to begin with optimism. I will get through the day with enthusiasm and a sense of purpose. I'll finish the day feeling fulfilled but not exhausted. I'm good enough and no one can be able to take my faith away from me. I am who I am and there isn't an equivalent.

Your daily affirmation may be whatever you would like to make it However, it should be motivating, it must be informative and real. It shouldn't be focused on the way your hair looks or how beautiful your clothes look. The focus should always be on your personal strengths not about your appearance. It is possible to change your mind anytime And putting all your trust in appearances and appearances will result in failure in the future.

Conclusion

I hope this book has helped examine the effects of stress and what is it able to do, and lastly, to provide you develop the right techniques to deal with stress. It's always a battle for anyone suffering from stress, but it's not something to be embarrassed about. It is crucial to have the strength to reach out to assistance because if you don't then the results are unacceptable. Recognizing the signs of stress earlier and showing the willingness and determination to get over it is vital. Don't let yourself be overwhelmed by sorrow and pain even though there is many things you can do to enhance your health and well-being. The book provided specific solutions and tips that I wish that you apply the knowledge you've gained to assist yourself and those around you.

www.ingramcontent.com/pod-product-compliance
Lightning Source LLC
Chambersburg PA
CBHW060334030426
42336CB00011B/1332